RAISING A CHILD WITH AUTISM

How to Cultivate Strength and Encouragement as a Parent

by Timothy Fountain

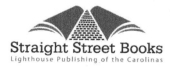

Straight Street Books
Lighthouse Publishing of the Carolinas

RAISING A CHILD WITH AUTISM – HOW TO CULTIVATE STRENGTH
AND ENCOURAGEMENT AS A PARENT
BY TIMOTHY FOUNTAIN
Published by Straight Street Books, an imprint of
Lighthouse Publishing of the Carolinas
2333 Barton Oaks Dr., Raleigh, NC, 27614

ISBN: 978-1-938499-38-8
Copyright © 2016 by Timothy Fountain
Cover design by Elaina Lee
Interior design by Karthick Srinivasan

Available in print from your local bookstore, online, or from the publisher at:
www.lighthousepublishingofthecarolinas.com.

For more information on this book and the author visit:
https://caregivingstinks.wordpress.com/

Brought to you by the creative team at Lighthouse Publishing of the Carolinas:
Eddie Jones, Kelsey Campbell, Cindy Sproles, and Shonda Savage.

Library of Congress Cataloging-in-Publication Data
Fountain, Timothy
*Raising a Child with Autism – How to Cultivate Strength and Encouragement
as a Parent*/Timothy Fountain 1st ed.

Printed in the United States of America

PRAISE FOR *RAISING A CHILD WITH AUTISM*
HOW TO CULTIVATE STRENGTH AND
ENCOURAGEMENT AS A PARENT

As a parent of a young adult with a disability, I could relate to many of Tim's stories. I found it so interesting how he was able to tell the story of raising Joey, all while teaching us Scripture. He reiterates how God is in control. I love how the story unfolds through the experience of the life of him and Melissa and their love for gardening. We nurture our children and fertilize our gardens. It all takes patience. Still, things may not develop the way we hope or plan. It shows that in all things, it is in God's plan, in his time and revealing God's love.

~ **Julie Briggs**
Human Rights Community Coordinator,
City of Sioux Falls, South Dakota

Tim Fountain's book is fascinating as he relates his dedication to the care of plant life. This is in parallel to the devotion and nourishment that he and his wife share for their autistic son. The use of applicable Scripture throughout the book is ingenious. This work is a masterpiece.

~**Brother Benet Tvedten, OSB**
Author of *How to Be a Monastic and Not Leave Your Day Job*;
The Motley Crew; *A View from a Monastery*

TABLE OF CONTENTS

Let's Dig In 1

I. Don' t Call Us 5

II. Not So Fast 9

III. Umm, That's Not What We Were Hoping For............13

IV. Skinny Sticks...17

V. Silver Roses 21

VI. Tomato Madness..25

VII. We're Being Followed..29

VIII. All Thumbs, No Green.......................................33

IX. Ice Storm 37

X. Ice Buds 41

XI. Tragic Beans 45

XII. Consider the Lilies of the Patio...........................49

XIII. Maybe Next Year 53

XIV. Annuals...57

XV. It Smells Good When You Try and Try Again............61

XVI. Scruffy Friends 65

XVII. They Are What They Eat? 69

XVIII. Sole Survivor 73

XIX. Talk Dirty..77

XX. Rocky Road 81

XXI. Forget Me Not..85

XXII. Out of Control 89

XXIII. Fire Ants! 93

XXIV. Sprinkler Blow Out and Whatever
the Opposite of That Is 97

XXV. The Evergreen..99

XXVI. A Moving Story 103

XXVII. With the Best of Intentions............................107

LET'S DIG IN

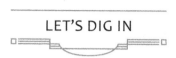

Melissa and I celebrated our 25th anniversary in 2015. One of the ongoing giggles of our marriage is due to our amateur effort to grow stuff. Fruits and veggies, trees, lawns, flowers, houseplants, you name it, we try it. We've had plenty of failures, but more often we have been blessed with fragrances, flavors, colors, and cover better than we imagined when we first got down to dig and plant.

Four years into our marriage, a different kind of seed was planted. We had our second son, Joseph. He was a perky little chap like his older brother Tim. The normal perky toddler behavior didn't seem to be kicking in.

He was diagnosed with autism, which the National Institute of Health defines as [1]"a range of complex neurodevelopment disorders, characterized by social impairments, communication difficulties, and restricted, repetitive, and stereotyped patterns of behavior." If you think our gardening was amateur hour, imagine our efforts to deal with that.

Maybe you don't have to imagine. Maybe you are an amateur trying to be caregiver, therapist, clinician, advocate, Mommy, Daddy, and everything else to a loved one living with autism. You feel like a lone idiot with a leaky hose when the job needs a landscape company. Or maybe you know someone else who is feeling fruitless, and you want to help out.

---

[1] National Institute of Neurological Disorders and Stroke, "Autism Fact Sheet," August 21, 2013 update

Whatever your reason for giving this book a look, Melissa and I hope that our tales of learn-as-you-go gardening and their application to raising an autistic kid will be useful to you. Sure, we have all kinds of ideas we think might help, but what we found out in our yards and gardens applies to all aspects of life: you learn by making the effort even when the end result isn't predictable.

And that's why we've included wisdom beyond ours in this book. We've matched our weed patch of stories and reflections with insight from the Word of God. When it comes to raising Joey, we've found the help of a better gardener who is patient and humble enough to work in the stinky dirt with us.

> Then he told this parable: "A man had a fig tree growing in his vineyard, and he went to look for fruit on it but did not find any. So he said to the man who took care of the vineyard, 'For three years now I've been coming to look for fruit on this fig tree and haven't found any. Cut it down! Why should it use up the soil?' "'Sir,' the man replied, 'leave it alone for one more year, and I'll dig around it and fertilize it. If it bears fruit next year, fine! If not, then cut it down.'" (Luke 13:6-9 NIV)

Jesus comes alongside us in our disappointments. He offers patience when we're fed up. He brings calm when our emotions storm. In some mysterious ways, he takes over when we give up. And with his special attention, beauty blooms. We watch Joey grow, and we delight in so much of who he is, both as an individual and as a blessing to us. He is a joy we couldn't have anticipated, like when a seed is planted and it finally blooms. And with Jesus' help, Joey's life is more abundant than our amateurism could have cultivated.

Each chapter of this book begins with a short account of our amateur gardening efforts where we will dig around to find a similar experience in raising a son with autism. Finally, we fertilize the experiences with reflections on that greater gardener: Jesus.

Each chapter stands on its own. We hope that some of them or all of them together provide that "special attention" you or someone you know needs for another season of caregiving.

Tim Fountain, a blooming idiot, October 2015

I. DON'T CALL US

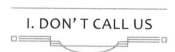

I had a nice apartment with a generous balcony when Melissa and I were dating. Purple is her favorite color, and I decided to beautify the balcony with some small potted trees that sported purple flowers. They looked great until the first wind blew the purple petals away. And they never came back.

Melissa is gracious enough to confess that she's no good with houseplants either. We've received plenty of them over time, as housewarming, anniversary, and other special occasion gifts. And we've made short work of most of them. Don't call us if you need your plants tended while you're on vacation.

If these plants could come back and sue us, there would be a formidable list of grievances:

- Long periods of neglect
- Near-drowning after extended neglect
- Abuse by burning with the latest magic chemical when trying to compensate for neglect
- Denial of shade to "grows best in shade" varieties
- Denial of sun to "grows best in sun" varieties
- Failure to read instructions
- Failure to ask competent people how to tend the plants

The simple fact is that we've had way better outcomes with our outdoor planting. Something about the houseplants eludes us. Our thumbs have a green glimmer outside but turn moldy and withered when we step indoors.

Digging Around

If our efforts to raise houseplants have been hit and miss, imagine some of the misadventures of raising a son with autism. Caregiving provides instant and constant experiences of inadequacy. Just as we've tried various strategies to keep the plants growing, we've sought out an array of therapies, settings, medications, specialists, diets and more to bring out the best in Joey's life. And even with all that help, there are plenty of withered efforts to report.

Some approaches failed and were abandoned. Others worked with a bit of adjustment, like moving a glum-looking potted plant into better sunlight to perk it up.

One example is the way Joey benefits from music therapy. Engaging him with songs and instruments increases his attention span, helps his motor skills, and, most of all, has him interacting purposefully with another person.

But we discovered that it has to be the right person. One music therapist was an excellent instrumentalist but had a limited vocal range. Joey knitted his brow and made I-just-bit-a-lemon lips every time the poor chap sang.

We eventually changed over to a therapist with a folk singing background, and Joey was quite pleased and made some amazing strides in attention span with her.

Caregiving is a constant encounter with limitations. It is important to admit failures without despair. Try again or, if the approach is proving fruitless, let it go and explore something new. Never be ashamed to seek help. Turn to someone else and say, "OK, this isn't working. Any ideas?"

In other words, if the thing in the flowerpot is brown, drooped over and crinkly, dump it out. Allow yourself a deep sigh, and then head back to the garden shop. Don't be shy about asking the garden pro lots of questions before you buy that new bag of potting soil and seeds.

Fertilizer

So, where does this Jesus, the great gardener, come into failures and do-overs? Many people think that Jesus' followers stand apart from life's struggles, judging those who do not rise to some religious idea of perfection. But the truth is that we have a profound sense of our own imperfection.

"Not that we are competent in ourselves to claim anything for ourselves, but our competence comes from God" (2 Corinthians 3:5 NIV).

Trying to bring beauty out of clay pots or bare earth is not something for which Melissa and I were naturally "competent." Other translations of that Bible verse use the words "adequate" or "sufficient." We had to confront our own inadequacy over and over as stuff failed to grow.

But beauty did grow when we resisted despair and accepted second, third, fourth, and more chances to try again. Had we allowed our own failures to shame us into giving up on gardening, we'd have been surrounded by dirt, rocks, and weeds. We had to accept the freedom to experience failures and take new chances, often with considerable help from others.

As caregivers, the stakes were even higher. Joey's health and happiness were more than wilted flowers to throw away. The sense of shame when some effort didn't benefit him was overwhelming. We were inadequate to his needs.

Which is exactly where the good gardener walked in. Our sufficiency was not in any preexisting set of skills and talents. Rather, it was that a good and loving God placed us in Joey's life. It didn't always feel like that because our emotions would grab onto our inadequacy. But we were sufficient because God gave us freedom to fail and try again. God led us into the freedom to set aside pride and ask others for help. We were sufficient because God loved Joey and assigned us as his caregivers.

Jesus, the good gardener, teaches us that, as insufficient as we might feel, his care for our lives and the lives placed in our care is sufficient. He tends fruitless trees and gives them new seasons in which to flourish.

II. NOT SO FAST

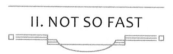

Our first flower bed was a delight. It was alongside a curving walkway to the front door of a brand-new house. We filled it with colorful flowers that said, "Welcome!" better than any doormat.

Weeds showed up, but it was easy just to pluck them up on my way to pick up the morning newspaper in the driveway. (Yes, this was way back when people had papers in their driveways instead of the latest little tech thingy for daily news. I wonder if you're reading this book on your toothbrush. But I digress.)

One morning, I noticed a big ugly weed. I don't know how it grew up without being detected. It was a raggedy, shaggy shock of vertical leaves, like zombie romaine lettuce.

Ticked off at this desecrator of the flower bed and how it had outwitted me long enough to grow into an eyesore, I stomped over to rip it out of the ground. Then I realized that it had concealed itself by growing right out of the root ball of a short flowering bush we'd planted. If I ripped out the weed, I risked hurting the good plant.

It was microsurgery, but I flicked away earth until I could find the weed's roots, disentangled them from the bush's roots, and lifted the nasty intruder out of the flower bed. It meant slowing down and taking a bit more time and effort, but our good plant came out the better for it.

Digging Around

Here's a selfish thought: Actually caring for Joey is a big

challenge to writing a book about caring for Joey. Things I'd like to do fall prey to things that need doing. And the things that need doing are for someone else, not for me. Me, myself, and I is the gross weed embedded in my family.

My comfort zone is time spent in quiet reflection. But uninterrupted, focused time is not something that caregiving favors. What I call "chore frenzies" are the norm. No matter how well we've organized the household, autism means unexpected loads of laundry due to "accidents," kitchen spills, bedding changes in the wee hours of the morning, appliances messed up by manic button-pushing, calendar mix-ups over medical and educational appointments, emotional outbursts to calm impromptu shopping runs for something Joey is willing to eat. These and many others often happen all at once or one right after another. It is like having a baby, except the baby stays a baby for a couple of decades.

In fact, I'm being yanked away from composing this chapter as we speak. Our son seems to have developed acid reflux or some other digestive system malady in the last few months. All of a sudden, he makes this awful gagging sound. It can't be ignored. It's loud and distressed enough that it could mean he's vomiting all over his room or having a major seizure. So I've had to stop writing at least three times to run in and check on him. Fortunately, he just needs an antacid.

But now my temper's up. The last time he gagged and broke my concentration, I didn't go to him. I just turned and spat out, "Joey, are you okay?" in a venomous tone that really said: "Will you just shut up?"

That's not caregiving. That's caregiving breaking down. Counting to ten and other simple life skills are necessary. Recognizing that some tasks and enjoyable activities will have to be put on hold is Caregiving 101. It means slowing down and rolling with imperfect situations. The weed and the flower grow close together, their roots sharing the same bit of earth. Sure, a violent tug can get rid of the weed, but it takes focused, patient effort to disentangle those roots without hurting the flower in the process.

Fertilizer

Taking care of a son who lives with autism exposes some ugly weeds in my heart. I find myself racing, but not in urgency to help Joey. There is a selfish urge to get his needs out of the way so I can get on with mine.

It is a spiritual challenge, one that Jesus takes time to address as he tends us and helps us to grow. He told a farming story to make the point: "'Do you want us to go and pull them up?' 'No,' he answered, 'because while you are pulling the weeds, you may uproot the wheat with them. Let both grow together until the harvest. At that time I will tell the harvesters: First collect the weeds and tie them in bundles to be burned; then gather the wheat and bring it into my barn'" (Matthew 13:28-30 NIV).

Jesus' little story about weed pulling answers a fundamental human question, "Why doesn't God just come fix all the bad stuff?"

His answer is that good and evil grow close together. If we are honest, we find good and evil roots entangled in our own hearts.

Jesus tells us that God is patient. God gives us time to let good fruit of the Holy Spirit flourish in our lives and to dig out our unholy thoughts and deeds— the "weeds" that choke our lives. God will not act abruptly because he loves us and wants to gather us into his "barn"—his heavenly kingdom. As one of his friends put it, "The Lord is not slow in keeping his promise, as some understand slowness. Instead he is patient with you, not wanting anyone to perish, but everyone to come to repentance" (2 Peter 3:9 NIV).

We have to recognize the great daily patience lavished on us by God. And as we become aware of this, we must, in turn, lavish that patience upon others, not trying to "pull out the weeds" with harsh or frantic reactions, but applying calm, steady, and delicate care to the aggravating, imperfect people around us.

III. UMM, THAT'S NOT WHAT WE WERE HOPING FOR

Marigolds graced the front walkway of our second house. You can be a blooming idiot, but the name sure sounds right. They're merry! They're gold! They are bright flowers that light up the world, and that's just what we wanted in our garden. So we planted marigolds. Lots of 'em. And they grew well and shed a joyful glow around our front door.

And they attracted bees. Lots of 'em. People walking to our door had to brave a gauntlet of them. We loved the marigolds, so they stayed. And so did the bees, although they were not what we were hoping for when we planted those flowers.

Digging Around

Joey is both marigolds and bees. We love him, and he's unusually emotionally connected and affectionate for a person with autism. He is a joy and delight in our lives. At the same time, autism brings stuff we'd love to do without.

One of the worst stings our family suffered was Joey's teenage onset of grand mal seizures. The first one came with no warning, and we thought we'd watched him die right in front of us. It is a sickening memory.

Although Joey's seizures are less frequent since he got past puberty's brain chemical chaos, one will sneak up on him now and then. The big danger is a head or neck injury from a fall.

Any loud noise will make us scramble to respond. I noticed my anxiety rising at a gym when the really big lifters dropped their massive weights at the end of a set. The kaboom of metal plates hitting the floor sounded too much like one of Joey's seizures in progress.

One night at home, Melissa heard a crash and rushed out of our bedroom to help Joey, only to find it wasn't Joey down. It was me. I'd gone to help Joey dry off after his bath and slipped on water he'd splashed out of the tub.

I was fine, but Joey's reaction wasn't what one might hope. He was laughing. I mean cracking up. To him, it was like a pratfall in a comedy. He thought I was doing something to entertain him. It was up to Melissa to say the right things like, "Are you OK?"

Such is life with autism. What you hope for often isn't what you get. We put our hearts into protecting Joey from falls, but we assumed that along with his physical safety we would be rewarded with his heart's appreciation and compassion. Instead, my dangerous tumble amused him.

Marigolds by your front door bring swarms of bees. You get lots of buzzing when you were hoping for company knocking.

Fertilizer

So, Jesus, great gardener, any advice for enjoying my marigolds with a swarm of bees around my head? "[Love] always protects, always trusts, always hopes, always perseveres" (1 Corinthians 13:7 NIV).

Hmmph. I was hoping for a spray that makes them go away. But the bees love the marigolds as much as I do, so I suppose love will bring them right back.

The philosopher Kierkegaard said that love is like a dash or hyphen. It is always out there seeking connection. God's description of love assumes that the connection won't always happen quickly or easily. So there's a need to maintain hope that it will come and to endure when it's missing.

Autism calls for this kind of love. You don't get what you expect. Autistic people don't play by all the social rules the rest of us figure out. There's very little "tit for tat" or "quid pro quo" because an autistic person is intensely directed from within, with little of the usual human reaction to the world.

Yet this can teach us to love with great depth. It challenges us to dig deep for a love that can endure without quick rewards and can "bear all things."

Of course, it can cut the other way as well. Loving an autistic kid can empty us out and exhaust us emotionally.

Yet even that presents an opportunity. It can open us up to the possibility of God, who loves us even when we don't love in return. In a spiritual sense, we're all "autistic." We are self-directed, self-absorbed beings who go through life without acknowledging or even recognizing the many blessings that come our way in every moment.

So is God feeling empty and exhausted from loving us? Not at all, and that's because God's love "always protects, always trusts, always hopes, always perseveres." If we can believe that, it might be that we can receive that. And in receiving God's inexhaustible love, we find ourselves better equipped to share it with those in our care no matter their response.

Can we see ourselves as God's marigolds? Can we believe that we are the "bee's knees" to God?

IV. SKINNY STICKS

We were the first homeowners in a freshly built tract. The floors were still bare concrete, the windows had no blinds or drapes, and the yard was just dirt.

We had to answer questions like, "Hydroseed or sod?" and "Berber or shag?" At least, we knew that we wanted the grass to be green. Oh, and we wanted some trees.

This was in our young, vigorous days, so rather than have a real landscaper plant some grown trees, we went and bought our own shovel, hose, and three small birches. Each was taped to a stick to help it stand up in its plastic bucket of dirt. They weren't much more than skinny sticks themselves.

The front yard soil was compacted during construction, which meant the house wouldn't sink, but it made the ground dense and hard to dig in. We managed to punch three holes in the ground and got the birch trees out of their buckets and into the earth. Then we ran the hose out and watered them abundantly because somewhere we heard that they could have "transplant shock" without an immediate drink.

They were the first trees either of us had planted. So we kept questioning the nursery, the neighbors, and anybody else unlucky enough to be in the path of our anxiety. We applied everything we heard. We got a funny little pipe to pinprick the yard so air could get to the roots. We watered the surface, and we forced "deep watering" below ground. We inspected the berms around the base of each tree to make sure they had a pool of water for their root balls.

One day, we realized that the supporting sticks were

hanging by their green tape. Though still skinny little things, our three birches were sturdy enough to stand tall without artificial support.

After we moved quite a distance away, we didn't pass by the house again for a few years. When a trip took us near the old neighborhood, we just had to have a look.

The three birches were magnificent and so tall that they were visible against the sky from blocks away. The new owners laid in ground cover and brickwork around them. Our skinny trees grew into the highlight of that whole street.

Digging Around

Like seeing the birch trees flourish from fragile beginnings, watching our son reach adulthood brings us satisfaction and even awe at results beyond what we had planned or guided. We didn't know he would have a sense of humor and certainly didn't coach him in comedy, but his ability to make others laugh is a quality noted by the staff of day programs he attends.

Several doctors praised us for our son's emotional connection, affection, and happiness. Those who live with autism, whatever they might feel within, are challenged in their ability to express it and seem aloof if not completely detached from the feelings of those around them. We didn't have special knowledge or strategy to cultivate Joey's warmth toward us. We just stayed close to him early on.

Melissa sang to him on days when he didn't seem to hear a note. Now as a young adult, he can enjoy an entire musical at the local playhouse. We pursued conversations with him even when he didn't make eye contact or walked away. Now he can attend social events even if he just stands smiling on the edge of the party. We made his place at the dinner table even when he had the habit of taking a bite and then running a repetitive pattern around the house. We would shrug and say, "Hate to eat and run." Now he eats in restaurants.

And, of course, there were teachers, therapists, and others who helped us care for Joey and who did their part to nurture his growth. Just as we needed advice to get the skinny birch trees planted, and they prospered with the folks who bought the house and did some special landscaping, Joey's life is so much better thanks to many caring people.

The professionals who observe Joey describe him as healthy and happy. Like the birches standing tall over the old neighborhood, that's a magnificent outcome from vulnerable, anxious beginnings.

Fertilizer

It doesn't matter if it's a birch tree or a baby; it needs help to grow. But none of us is enough to give a growing life all that it needs. Those skinny birch trees were planted by novice gardeners, after all. Thank goodness there were landscapers and others with advice.

Raising Joey taught us to do our part, accept our limitations, and thankfully receive help others could give. Most of all, we learned that we couldn't possibly be all things that Joey needed, but that Joey was in the care of Jesus, the great gardener who could bring all kinds of great folks together to help our son grow.

"What, after all, is Apollos? And what is Paul? Only servants, through whom you came to believe—as the Lord has assigned to each his task. I planted the seed, Apollos watered it, but God has been making it grow. So neither the one who plants nor the one who waters is anything, but only God, who makes things grow" (1 Corinthians 3:5-7 NIV).

Each of us is a gift from God to the world. Each of us brings some unique quality, skill, or wisdom that blesses others' lives. But no one of us is the whole blessing.

That's the way Jesus tends and nurtures life. He brings together the right people at the right time in a marvelous plan. We can see our part, but we only have glimpses of the whole effort. But when the results become plain over time, like when we saw the birch trees touching the sky or when we get goofed on by one of Joey's affectionate jokes, our hearts swell with wonder and gratitude.

It is both humbling and beautiful to recognize that our

little contributions are part of a bigger assortment of blessings that Jesus assembles to grow a life. None of us can be everything another person needs, but we can be the right ingredient at the right moment as God nurtures that person toward eternal glory.

As caregivers, there is inner peace in the knowledge that we are not responsible for everything. We can't possibly control all the details of a life, for good or for ill. God, who is the source, keeper, and ultimate destination of all life, doesn't expect that of us.

But we are far from irrelevant. Jesus makes us part of God's eternal work. There are skinny sticks that need planting and a lifetime of help if they are to reach up high.

V. SILVER ROSES

One year, my wife and I planted roses all around our backyard. If we knew what we were doing, we would tell you that the flowers were called *Lady Wilhelmina Sunburst Spectaculars* or some such name. The reality is we went to the nursery and said things like, "Oh, let's get some of those silver ones."

Sure, we had red roses and yellow roses, but we were really excited by the bush that would give us silver roses. Our friends would stare and sputter, "Wow, *silver* roses. Never seen those."

We planted the silver rose bush in a prominent angle of our fence line. It would be the eye-catching star of the backyard. We followed the nursery's instructions about how deep to dig, how much to water, and whether it liked red or white wine with meals.

Our dog at the time was a burly malamute mix named Rocky. Evidently, he shared our interest in silver roses. We came home one afternoon to find Rocky lying on the grass, gnawing on the dug-up silver rose bush.

After much arm-flapping and loud shouts of, "Oh no!" and "Bad dog!" we replanted the bush. It was battered but not devoured. The root ball was intact since Rocky ignored that like parsley on a dinner plate.

I wish we could brag that we sat with the rose bush in 24-hour shifts in snow, heat, and wildebeest stampedes, or that we applied some newfound expertise in plant rehab. All we did was stick it back in the hole and put the dirt back around it. Rocky was a good dog and left it alone.

A few weeks later, we had our silver roses. We were

impressed that a lovely plant was hearty enough to survive dog teeth and amateur gardeners.

Digging Around

That rose bush didn't pout because a couple of beginning gardeners forgot to protect it from their dog. It just went back to making silver roses.

Our son Joey endured much because his caregivers were medical amateurs. We never spotted warning signs before a seizure caused him to bang his head on a TV stand, making him bleed profusely. He couldn't tell us that a stomach bug had him dehydrated, and all we could do was watch the emergency room nurses give him an IV to re-inflate him like a tire.

But after incidents like those, he just took up wherever he left off. Our expertise—or lack thereof—didn't bother him. He went back to his daily routines and loved us just the same.

Joey is not what we made him or failed to make him. He's always carried strengths of his own that we can admire as precious gifts from God.

Fertilizer

We underestimated the hardiness of that silver rose bush, and we often took upon ourselves too much anxiety about Joey, assuming that he was all fragility and no stability. We are part of a culture that takes responsibility for too much and assumes that our every word, deed, or thought will have a life altering impact (usually for the worse). Caregivers take that warped thinking to another level since we are in constant interaction with people who have special needs, and we assume that we will do them more harm by our perceived failures.

We need to stop and examine those thoughts. What if those around us "are who they are," no matter what we do or don't do?

"For we are to God the pleasing aroma of Christ among those who are being saved and those who are perishing. To the one we are an aroma that brings death; to the other, an aroma that brings life. And who is equal to such a task?" (2

Corinthians 2:15-16 NIV).

We are who we are. Others are who they are, too. Our impact on them is dictated as much by their own inner workings as by our intention and skill. The silver rose bush was going to grow silver roses in spite of our amateurish tending. Joey was going to bounce back from emergencies because he's resilient without us having to teach him resilience.

I think we can find some freedom and peace in what the Apostle Paul blurts out, "And who is equal to such a task?" Well, I'm not. You? So let's drop fear of failure from the one hand and fantasy futures from the other and concentrate on taking hold of what is true in the relationships entrusted to us by God in the here and now. Those placed in our care have special needs we can meet, but they are unique people and not just extensions of our lives. Silver roses are not our creations; they are the beautiful flowers of tough plants.

VI. TOMATO MADNESS

Why do we use the phrase "throwing rotten tomatoes" when, in fact, most people throw perfectly good ones around? Not literal tossing and splattering, mind you, but stuffing them into grocery bags to pitch at someone, anyone, who will take them.

Tomatoes are fruit that even the most inexperienced gardener can grow. It's getting them to *stop* growing that requires skill.

We grew some in pots on the tiny patio of our Southern California duplex. We had these cone-shaped metal cages stuck in the pots to help the plants grow vertically. Instead, the vines crawled up the frames, popped the frames out of the soil and tossed them aside. Then the green invaders spread out to take over the patio and fill it with their admittedly tasty fruit.

The eatin' was good, but after awhile we desired fewer tomato slices for sandwiches, salads, and salsa blends. That's when the throwing started.

Several full bags wound up in a break room at work. Some landed in the fellowship hall at church. Our coworkers, friends, and neighbors were confronted by grocery bags of tomatoes, and perky "Take all you want!" signs gleaming at them from the shiny plastic bags.

But while we were throwing our tomatoes to the four winds, the four winds were throwing them right back at us. Our coworkers, friends, and neighbors grew tomatoes of their own. Pretty soon, our doorstep sported bulging plastic bags with smiley faces and "Enjoy!" written in giant permanent marker.

Then it was time to share zucchini.

Digging Around

The art of caregiving includes finding enjoyable activities for the people in our care. I get a surge of satisfaction when I come up with something that brightens our son's day. If he's calm and happy, we find *ourselves* a bit closer to calm and happy.

The downside is that the good times can sprawl like tomato plants. An autistic person, for example, can impose constant demands for the feel-good activity. Our bedroom door flies open and light floods in at 2 a.m. because Joey wants that video that made him laugh throughout the day. It is a short step from "Thank God, I've found something he likes," to "Please, God, make him stop bugging me about that."

Joey's love of Christmas is another good thing that gets overgrown. Since moving to South Dakota and feeling the change of seasons, he's learned to anticipate it with considerable accuracy.

The downside is that he mimics the department stores that put up Christmas displays like overgrown tomato cages from about October on. As soon as autumn leaves drop, he begins a constant repetition of statements like "Soon there will be presents" and "Working for presents," which translates as "My behavior will meet the minimum requirements for you to owe me a reward." In all fairness, that line of thought is due to years of "reinforcers" (items or activities given to people with autism to help them drop unwanted behaviors).

We tried to get rid of the repetition by planting a new thought. Every time he said "Working for presents," we said, "No work. Presents come because we love you."

As a reinforcer, love was no replacement for loot. We're still getting bagfuls of "Working for presents." We're glad he loves Christmas, but hearing about it all day and night through the fall and winter gets as tiresome as a daily diet of BLTs, salads, and salsa.

Fertilizer

We are not farmers nor do we play them on television. We're just gardeners with too many tomatoes. But here in the Midwest, we live in an agricultural setting, and we hear about things like "crop rotation." If you keep growing the same thing over and over on the same land, the land eventually runs out of chemicals and nutrients, and that particular crop won't grow anymore.

So the farmers give the ground some rest by growing a different crop every so often. Farmers will use a field that has produced corn for several seasons to grow soybeans or sunflowers. The nutrients that the corn needs are replenished and corn can come back on that land in the future.

We all need rest and recovery, even when our efforts are fruitful. Jesus is responsive to this reality of our human nature. "The apostles gathered around Jesus and reported to him all they had done and taught. Then, because so many people were coming and going that they did not even have a chance to eat, he said to them, 'Come with me by yourselves to a quiet place and get some rest'" (Mark 6:30-31 NIV).

We're not built to keep doing things—even good things—without breaks for rest and refreshment. We call it "respite" in caregiver jargon. The Bible speaks of "Sabbath." It's what Jesus wants for his people, and it imitates the rest taken by God after he shaped the life-giving order of which we're all a part.

God-given rest has the practical benefit of recharging our run-down energy and refilling our empty emotional tank. But more than that, it can transform our thinking and feelings. To take Sabbath time, we have to accept that the universe, both as a whole and in its littlest parts, doesn't depend upon us. We have to relax in the reality that God loves it and nurtures it—and us.

God assigns each person special work in his world, but every job comes with generous breaks and vacation. God wants us to take them.

VII. WE'RE BEING FOLLOWED

Our first house was in a densely populated, hot, and smoggy L.A. suburb. The next was in a quiet small town nestled between a forested mountain range and the desert. Then we moved to one of those Southern California developments where somebody pumped a bunch of water into an almost-desert and built a town on it. From there, we headed down toward the ocean in San Juan Capistrano, not right on the water but close enough that the late afternoon sea breeze was our air conditioner.

As I write this, we're in South Dakota, where a weekly church class commenced on an August night with temperatures and humidity both near 100. Then two months later, we had to postpone its final session due to a blizzard. And in all of these settings, with all their varieties of climate and terrain, we've had a steady but unwelcome presence: weeds.

They climbed the backyard fence in smoggy L.A. They snuck in among seasonal flowers in our pretty foothill garden. They found spots in the puny patios of the planned community and the house near the sea.

And in South Dakota? They show up among the first signs of spring, and they are still around when the leaves turn for fall. And the summers? Don't get me started. The heavy humidity and excruciating heat wilt man and beast, but the cornfields thrive, and the weeds are like German tourists carpeting Spanish beaches.

At least they stop bothering us in the winter. Pulling weeds for three-quarters of the year is a hated chore. It gets worse as I age. When I realize that my autistic kid is a physically healthy young man sitting in the air-conditioned house watching videos because weeding is too demanding for his attention span and underdeveloped fine motor skills, it is almost more than I can stand. Caregiving provides many such middle-age rip-offs.

Anyway, back to the weeds. In the height of summer, I can be pulling them daily. I can't ignore them too much because some are "stranglers," growing in among good plants and killing them. And summers here afford daylight until 9 p.m. So saying "It's getting dark" is not a viable excuse to stop.

You know what? Sometimes I don't make an excuse. I just say "no." I look ahead on the calendar for a day with a few open hours and write in the word "weeds." I make an appointment to see them. They're always in a hurry to arrive, but they're surprisingly indifferent about how often we interact. In fact, I get the feeling they would rather just go on about their business without me.

Digging Around

I was more on top of weed-pulling in our first garden, of course. I had the energy of youth, the pride of a new homeowner, and it seemed urgent. Likewise, in the early years of Joey's life, we were young enough to run ourselves ragged trying to do everything: work on every skill and learning drill, coach him through every small task, try to keep him engaged, clean up after him, visit and consult every expert, and go to every seminar and meeting.

As each year passed, we accepted more freedom just to say "no." We bore down on fruitful things that seemed to reach him, and we let go of things that didn't, even if it meant accepting defeat in some area of his life we wanted to improve.

We accepted that there would be all kinds of needs and issues all the time. This was true no matter how hard we worked and no matter how often we stepped back and dabbled in the rest of life.

We also learned more about depending upon others. I pay

friends' kids to pull my weeds these days. In raising a person with autism, there are free services and activities out in the community, and some for which you have to pay. Either way, there are good and competent folks who can enrich the life of a person who lives with autism. Music therapy, horseback riding, day camps, special needs sports groups like Special Olympics, and many others provide help with developmental progress and just plain fun and friendship. (Not to mention a breather for the exhausted caregiver.)

Fertilizer

You can spend all of your time pulling weeds. You'll have a nicer garden, a sore back, and a growing sense of futility. The job is never done.

An important foundation of life, and an acute issue for caregivers, is to know that our human worth is a gift from our Creator rather than something we earn by handling everything all the time. Jesus knew that he could spend every moment on a world full of need. He is, in fact, the ultimate caregiver; his life's mission was to give himself for others. Yet he accomplished his work by decisive action at key moments rather than constant frantic activity. In fact, he withdrew from action on a regular basis. "Very early in the morning, while it was still dark, Jesus got up, left the house and went off to a solitary place, where he prayed" (Mark 1:35 NIV).

Caregiving is holy work. But it is draining, exhausting, and always there.

Jesus, the one who cares for all of creation, poured his life out as a sacred offering on our behalf. But while accomplishing this, he would steal away to refresh himself in prayer.

Like Jesus, we need time to retreat from all of life's "weed pulling" and go into the presence of God. We need to connect with the One who is permanent among all the passing things of life. We need to breathe deeply and be refilled by the source of life. Human caregivers need the divine Caregiver.

In prayer, we can be still and savor the love that is not based on what we do but based on who God is and what he's done to make us his own. In prayer, we are reminded that we are the recipients of great care, and the one who provides it has love, energy, and patience without limits.

VIII. ALL THUMBS, NO GREEN

A Mexican restaurant we enjoy makes guacamole right at your table. The waitress brings a whole avocado to scoop, squash, and mix it with seasoning into tasty green dip. They have a special bag in which they put the big brown avocado pit, so you can take it home and grow an avocado of your own. The instructions are printed right on the bag.

Melissa and I took a seed home, poked in some toothpicks to suspend it over a glass of water, and went to bed to dream of a guacamole-made-from-scratch party in our very own kitchen.

Things didn't go so well. Instead of wispy roots growing down into the water, there was a thick white thing, like a tusk, growing from the bottom of the seed.

Up top, spindly fibers poked up and then lolled over, like the meager hair on the top of my head.

We kept going back to the little paper bag from the restaurant, obsessing over the instructions like it was Christmas morning and we had a "some assembly required" toy for an impatient kid.

We never got our homegrown avocado. Apparently, we'd set the seed upside down.

Digging Around

Even with simple instructions on the package, we proved ourselves inexperienced idiots with that avocado pit. Imagine the challenges for families living with autism, who are bombarded with advice like: Try this medical treatment, that therapeutic method, the other diet, a new medicine, or stop using some medical, therapeutic, nutritional, or pharmacological approach. And do it right now.

I guess it can't be any other way. There is no magic cure for autism. You have to take in lots of advice and experiment with different approaches because what lifts the life of one autistic kid could be fruitless or even counterproductive with another.

The universal manual of "normal" parenting, like the avocado seed instructions on the carry out bag, fails to help. Normal parenting is to yell if you spot an emergency in progress. But if we'd raised our voices and warned Joey, "Hey, put that down. You'll put your eye out," we'd be living with a Cyclops by now. You learn to use soft, reassuring tones to say, "Honey, you're standing in front of an oncoming bus there. How about standing with Mommy instead?"

You find yourself looking at the world upside down. That position isn't good for avocado pits, but caregivers and people living with autism have to work from that position.

Fertilizer

The good news is that you can be upside down and just fine with God. Some of Jesus' better-known words point this out, but we tend to hear them as beautiful phrases to cross-stitch and display rather than radical words by which to live.

> And Jesus opened his mouth and taught them, saying: "Blessed are the poor in spirit, for theirs is the kingdom of heaven. Blessed are those who mourn, for they shall be comforted. Blessed are the meek, for they shall inherit the earth. Blessed are those who hunger and thirst for righteousness, for they shall be satisfied. Blessed are the merciful, for they shall receive mercy. Blessed are the pure in heart, for they shall see God. Blessed are the peacemakers, for they shall be called sons of God. Blessed are those who are persecuted for righteousness' sake, for theirs is the kingdom

of heaven. Blessed are you when others revile you and persecute you and utter all kinds of evil against you falsely on my account. Rejoice and be glad, for your reward is great in heaven, for so they persecuted the prophets who were before you. (Matthew 5:2-12 NIV)

In one of my favorite lessons on these words, the preacher had a young gymnast come up from the congregation and maintain a handstand while he spoke:

"Blessed means 'happy.' It's happy to be sad? It's happy to feel empty or fall short of a goal? It's happy to have people ignore you except to say mean things about you? This is all upside down. Just like our friend doing the handstand here. She sees the room from a completely different point of view."

The life of faith challenges us to be upside down. Out of step. Not ready for prime time. Fashion disasters.

But there is no simple manual for raising someone who lives with autism. Caregiving often involves going against "normal" ways of doing things. Jesus tells us that being upside down like that is how we learn to see eye-to-eye and heart-to-heart with the invisible God above, beside and within us, and that this God can help us see eye-to-eye and heart-to-heart with the mystery of autism.

IX. ICE STORM

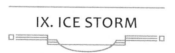

One morning in April 2013, I was picking up my car keys to head for work when the sky went nighttime-dark and all of the north facing windows of our house clouded with ice. It was like watching time-lapse photography. An ice storm jumped on Sioux Falls, South Dakota.

How bad was it? Well, for the first time in eight years of trying to be South Dakotans, we kind of qualified. It was the first time that the real South Dakotans couldn't say, "Oh, that was nothing. You should have been here for the big storm of '08." None of the folks in Sioux Falls remembered anything like the ice storm of '13.

Nasty as it was, it didn't hurt our garden plants. They slept through it, still dormant from the winter. Missing the whole thing, they roused themselves a few weeks later to point spindly branches at the mess and ask one another, "What happened around here?"

It was the trees that suffered. The ice built up on limbs, and it became unsafe to go outside as the weight snapped and dropped them. For days the air was filled with groans, cracks and crashes as trees sagged, limbs and even trunks snapped, and pieces or even whole trees smashed down on streets, cars and houses.

A neighbor's disintegrating tree kept beating against our house right by our bedroom. The scraping and pounding of swaying and breaking limbs kept us in constant anxiety. No matter how many times the tree debris didn't come through the wall, for days, it sounded like it was about to.

Our black lab Lily was so stressed that she threw up anything she ate.

We lost power for the better part of a day, and we were among the lucky ones. Some neighborhoods lost power for a week or more.

Not being true South Dakotans, we didn't have things like chainsaws sitting around. All I could muster was a hatchet. I hacked away with that for hours, breaking up limbs that leaned on our house and blocked the way to our front door.

The one tree trimmer we knew was tied up with emergencies. "The houses with trees through their roofs have to come first," was his reply to my frantic call for help. We wound up hiring a team from the hordes of out-of-state crews that drove in and cruised the city looking for cleanup work. The young Minnesotans clambered up our big maple and a couple of other trees to lop off threatening limbs and bring the chunks down safely.

We were thankful that none of our trees fell or had to be entirely cut down, but we had to get used to them being lopsided and not casting all the shade they used to.

The city directed people to pile up the debris along the curbs so that big side-loading trucks could come and haul it away. It took days, but the city did a magnificent job getting things back to something like normal.

We found out that we had made national and even international news. Our ice storm was a full-fledged disaster. It took over our lives for days and occupied much of our city's attention and efforts for months.

At least our trees looked suitably creepy for Halloween.

Digging Around

Our city's ice storm disaster takes place in miniature by way of autism's many household disasters. Taking care of Joey involves what I call "chore frenzies." His needs can turn into a storm of stuff that takes over the day. There are the usual household tasks, and then the kid has a bathroom accident or worse.

What do I mean by worse? Well, after doing a robust bit of laundry one Saturday, we had all of Joey's clothes clean, folded, and put away for the coming week. Then Joey didn't make it to the toilet in time and created a nasty lake on his bathroom floor. He took off the clothes he was wearing and tried to mop it up.

Then he needed a change. So he went to the chest of drawers in his room and took out a fresh set of clothes, but he also took the soaked clothing off of the bathroom floor and put that in the drawer full of freshly cleaned clothing. We had to start the laundry marathon all over, plus figure out how to deodorize the drawer. And there was still a bathroom to clean.

Raising a kid with autism can be as anxiety-provoking, frustrating and grinding as dealing with the ice storm. A completed task is replaced with another need, and another, and another ...

In the usual order of things, people who live with autism don't qualify for residential placement until age 21. So the parents of a special needs kid can be in a chore frenzy for two decades.

Joey's combination of great need and low participation is both heartbreaking and backbreaking for us. We have a young adult son who can't help rake the fall leaves, pick up after the pets, do dishes, or much of anything beyond picking up his room once in a blue moon. He can't slow the chore frenzy; he only revs it up. Sometimes physically, but more often emotionally, caregivers sag like the ice-burdened trees. We wonder if our groaning means we're bending with the effort or if it's the prelude to falling down.

Fertilizer

Ice storms and chore frenzies, disasters great and small, get our adrenaline pumping and convince us that they must be dealt with right now, ahead of anything else.

For example, it is my intention to start each day in prayer. But pans and dishes in the sink, an overflowing laundry hamper, or any number of other "priorities" can get me thinking, "If I just get those out of the way, the rest of the day will be easier. I'll be more focused when I pray, too."

Of course, the opposite happens. The day starts out as an unsatisfying rampage of unpleasant tasks, and beneficial things get rushed or ignored altogether. Prayer, conversation with family, exercise, preparing healthy food, and other actions that could bless the coming day are missed because of worry-driven attention to other "urgencies."

Jesus says that turning toward the eternal kingdom first will allow God to bring all of the temporary things we worry about into order. "But seek first his kingdom and his righteousness, and all these things will be given to you as well" (Matthew 6:33 NIV).

I find this proven again and again. If I start the morning in prayer, there seems to be plenty of time for all of the other stuff. Improved energy, focus, and serenity emerge. The clock seems to move at a friendlier pace. There's satisfaction instead of frenzy in knocking the tasks down one by one and less agitation when new ones come up.

And sometimes prayer is where I discover the peace of mind that says, "Slow down. The world won't end if you let some chores hang until later."

X. ICE BUDS

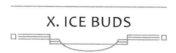

In winter, everything except the big evergreen in our yard goes bare and dormant. Unless snow comes to pretty it up, everything is brown or gray.

Some South Dakotans put what can only be described as bowling-ball-sized marbles on front yard pedestals for winter color. But the first time we saw those, Melissa and I looked at each other and shook our heads. We don't do the marbles.

When the big ice storm of 2013 hit, we were at the tail end of winter. There wasn't any snow, just brown lawns and gray trees. Oh, and there was all the limbs, branches, and trunks that the storm brought down.

But the ice storm produced some nice lawn decor, too.

The fallen tree parts were coated with ice. It was evenly applied, smooth, clear as glass and, even though this ice had snapped our trees apart, it was pretty.

Melissa noticed the most hypnotic feature of our new debris garden. Some of the branches of a honey locust tree were anticipating spring and had small magenta buds forming. These dots were ensconced in the pure ice from the sky, like candies coated in a shimmering glaze.

It wasn't what we wanted for our trees or our yard, but some of these natural ice sculptures actually reduced the anxiety of looking outside after the storm.

Digging Around

The beauty of the ice buds wasn't decor that we thought up or desired for our front yard. Nor did we sign up to have an autistic kid. I'm sure there are some awesome souls who've adopted a special needs person into their family, but the majority of us didn't choose our kids' special needs or the decades of caregiving that come with them.

And still, moments of great joy and beauty arrive with all the havoc. Laughter, in particular, bursts out at unexpected times. We had a prominent clergyman over for dinner, and our son came strolling into the dining room without any pants. It lightened up what might have been a very formal evening.

Things that are commonplace with "normal" kids are like miracles with an autistic child. A flash of empathy, like Joey knotting up his brow in realization that his behavior has hurt one of us, is cause for celebration, and the hurt is forgotten. A sentence instead of a grunt, or a peck on Mommy's cheek instead of a head butt, things like these are like getting that million-dollar inheritance from the crazy uncle you never knew you had.

In a life situation that we just fell into (or that fell on us), glorious beauty shows up, magnified because beauty is the last thing we expect.

Fertilizer

Caregivers and those in our care are like those ice buds. Caregivers are beautiful in the midst of situations that the world sees as messed up. Those in our care surprise us with beauty even as they diverge from our normal definitions of what's attractive and pleasant.

"You did not choose me, but I chose you and appointed you so that you might go and bear fruit—fruit that will last— and so that whatever you ask in my name the Father will give you" (John 15:16 NIV).

With all of our human imperfections, failures, compromises, and our sins, the perfect God chooses us. Amid the debris of our life's hurts, both things inflicted upon us and those we inflict upon ourselves and others, Jesus comes to call our names and let us share his holy work of restoring the universe to its original, unblemished beauty. Caregiving is part of his work.

We did not choose Jesus, but he chose us. And he looks at us and sees glorious beauty as we accept the caregiving work he's entrusted to us in the midst of challenges and chaos. We are glimmers of light and color in seemingly broken and barren situations.

XI. TRAGIC BEANS

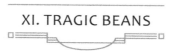

Melissa doesn't like doing things "just because." She has the need to know why. And amateur gardening means reading lots of instructions. "Do this, at this time, in this way," said the tiny little words on the seed packet. That's not Melissa's style. She wants to know why it should be done, why the particular time is important, and why it can't be done in a way that makes better sense to her. But the packets stare back in cold silence.

We lived in a place that felt like the country, so we decided to grow some food. One of our crops was green beans, except the beans came up purple. I had nowhere to hide when Melissa wanted to know why. In fact, I still don't know. I can't do much better than say, "I guess they're the purple kind."

But what really stressed Melissa were the instructions to plant the seeds in groups of three, then pluck out every third green sprout that would appear.

She recounts the experience, saying, "Killing this new life was horrendous. And it made me angry. Why was I supposed to bring a seed to life and pull it out of the ground?"

Still no good answer. I mean, we knew to pull weeds out so they wouldn't suck up all the resources needed by the good plants. But if three beans are a crowd, why not plant just two? But we followed the instructions.

And we did grow a nice little patch of beans, and we felt like legitimate farmers when we were able to collect them and serve them with meals. The health of the beans depended upon thinning out the plants, just like some flowers grow best when pruned.

But that knowledge just left us in a sour mood about having to rough up what we were trying to raise. We just had to get on with snipping and plucking.

Digging Around

People who live with autism practice "self-stimulating" behaviors to connect to the world around them. Known as "stimming," the actions are repetitive and are often the way the outside world recognizes someone as autistic.

Our son Joey has a callous on one knuckle from years of tapping his hand against his teeth. There were times when his hand or his mouth bled from the constant contact.

His button-pushing on TVs, VCRs, and DVD players drove us nuts. We spent all kinds of money on them as if they were consumable supplies.

The thing is, stimming is a calming, settling activity for an autistic person. Without it, anxiety revs up and tantrums, or even violent meltdowns, result. So caregivers have to learn the art of "redirection": finding some other stimming that isn't a danger to people or stuff.

Joey's safer stim involved waving things around. These became known as his "fidgets." Twisted up plastic bags worked. So did wiggly toys like a Slinky, as long as one didn't mind them being abused beyond all ability to slink. Crumpled pieces of paper were great for several years, but we had to hide targets of opportunity like bills and other important papers we didn't want him to stim on.

Helping him grow meant taking away things that he liked. It wasn't a happy experience for him or us at the time. But it produced a better quality of life for Joey and for those who share life with him.

Fertilizer

Plucking some early beans made for an abundant and tasty harvest later. But those "third beans" didn't get to be part of the harvest. They had to go so the other ones would grow well. Some items and habits that Joey enjoyed had to be plucked out of his daily behavior. Upsetting Joey in the short term by taking away his "stims" made for better behavior and more meaningful interaction with the world around him in the long run. We did not enjoy plucking the beans or plucking out the stims.

All people deal with having familiar things plucked out of our lives. And many of us suffer with minds and emotions conditioned to regard such uncomfortable experiences as punishments. I would be rich if I had a dollar for every time I moaned, "What did I do to deserve this?" The hurts and frustrations of caregiving can feel quite literally "like hell," a state of hopelessness and affliction imposed by God for the sins our minds (or a demon on our shoulder) keep bringing to memory.

But Jesus tells us that those who are loved by God and who are doing holy work—bearing fruit—will be "pruned." We will suffer unpleasant experiences on the way to growth. Jesus said, "I am the true vine, and my Father is the gardener. He cuts off every branch in me that bears no fruit, while every branch that does bear fruit he prunes so that it will be even more fruitful" (John 15:1-2 NIV).

We are prone to think that pleasure is always a blessing and pain is always a curse. But Jesus says that those loved by God will have the stuff that seemed essential taken away. We'll be deprived of things that brought us pleasure and relief, and more challenges will intrude on our lives.

Jesus assures us that this attention from God is not a punishment, but a loving effort to make us grow and thrive. Once when I threw a grand pity party over some problems, a wise friend said to me, "I think what's happening is that the old Tim has to die so that the new Tim can be born."

It takes some imagination, a new way of thinking, and a big leap of faith, but if you're someone who sees your struggles as God's punishment or indifference, try taking a moment in prayer. Say, "God, show me what Jesus means. What's the good fruit you are growing in my life by all of this pruning?"

Caregiving can be like reading the instruction to pluck

that third purple bean. Like Melissa, we want to know why. "What's the point?" But we go through with it even while our questions hang in the air. We take the steps, even though we hate it when we have to displease those in our care, and we hate it when their needs pluck familiar pleasures from our lives.

Jesus doesn't condemn us or give up on us for questioning. He knows that what we are going through is unpleasant and confusing, which is why he compares it to being snipped with a sharp tool. He asks us only to stay connected to him so that he can work through us. We endure uncertainties and suffer some losses so that those in our care can thrive as Jesus makes use of our inadequate blooming idiocy on their behalf. And as they grow, we discover new pleasures and rewards greater than our losses.

XII. CONSIDER THE LILIES OF THE PATIO

We grew some nice calla lilies in the little patio planter beds at one of the smaller houses we shared. They weren't exactly Easter lilies, but they grew right around Easter, and they made our little place feel special in that sacred season.

Joey liked them because they had long stalks and made perfect fidget toys. So he would rip up our pretty flowers and wave them around. Despite his lack of fine motor skills, he figured out how to unlatch and slide the patio door so he could go out and thrash our plants.

"If only he could use his powers for good," was the only gallows humor I could muster.

Digging Around

Joey has taught us a lot about saying goodbye to things we valued and enjoyed. We had a set of stoneware mugs from the bed-and-breakfast where we honeymooned. He threw one and shattered it.

We kept a little mesh bag of Jordan almonds from a place setting at our wedding reception. He ate them. Twenty years after the wedding.

We like watching movies together. But we can't keep a DVD player in our room because he'll either push buttons until it breaks or keep barging into our room demanding to use it. Speaking of barging into our room, we've lost count of the times he's denied us other private enjoyments of marriage.

We gave up on taking vacations that required long travel or extended stays away from home. Okay, no more examples.

I'm getting depressed remembering them all.

Fertilizer

We ached at the destruction of our lilies and lots of other pleasures he took from us over the years. But our love for Joey was always greater. He is our child, and he has needs and challenges beyond what life typically brings. We get frustrated from time to time, but our hearts always come back to him.

There's a disturbing incident in the reports of Jesus' life, and it makes sense only if we can appreciate the value of every troubled (and troubling) person.

> A large herd of pigs was feeding there on the hillside. The demons begged Jesus to let them go into the pigs, and he gave them permission. When the demons came out of the man, they went into the pigs, and the herd rushed down the steep bank into the lake and was drowned. When those tending the pigs saw what had happened, they ran off and reported this in the town and countryside, and the people went out to see what had happened. When they came to Jesus, they found the man from whom the demons had gone out, sitting at Jesus' feet, dressed and in his right mind; and they were afraid. Those who had seen it told the people how the demon-possessed man had been cured. Then all the people of the region of the Gerasenes asked Jesus to leave them, because they were overcome with fear. So he got into the boat and left. (Luke 8:32-37 NIV)

It's an unsettling story. People who go to the Bible for lovely words get turned off by this one. Those poor pigs, after all.

But it shows us how valuable every human being is to God. The healing of one crazy, scary guy on the outskirts of town was worth more than a whole herd of pigs. Those who had lost their property in the lake didn't appreciate their neighbor sitting there at peace after so many years of torment; they just wanted Jesus to get lost because of the mess he'd made while making the guy better.

Taking care of one off-the-wall, scary child of God means that a bunch of our nice stuff will get trashed. Pretty things, pleasant things, pricey things all take a beating when we take care of someone with autism or some other special need.

We can go down with our things and drown in a lake of resentment. Or we can find the love in our hearts that makes the well-being of that one person worth all the losses.

More than this, if we open our eyes of faith, we can see God's love for us. Jesus didn't just let the pigs drown; he became like them on his cross. Just as the pigs died so that the demon-infested man could be "clothed and in his right mind," Jesus died bearing our sins so that we would be clothed with new life.

Again and again, the Bible teaches that Jesus considered anything and everything worth losing to help us discover God's great love for us. "For you know the grace of our Lord Jesus Christ, that though he was rich, yet for your sake he became poor, so that you through his poverty might become rich" (2 Corinthians 8:9 NIV).

This included suffering and humiliation, such as caregivers experience while we love and care for people who seem unresponsive much of the time.

"But he was pierced for our transgressions, he was crushed for our iniquities; the punishment that brought us peace was on him, and by his wounds we are healed. We all, like sheep, have gone astray, each of us has turned to our own way; and the LORD has laid on him the iniquity of us all" (Isaiah 53:5-6 NIV).

XIII. MAYBE NEXT YEAR

Growing up in L.A., I was a fan of the Los Angeles Angels when they were a brand-new American League expansion team. This was before they built their own stadium down in Anaheim. When I was a kid, they played in the stadium named for the "real" team: the Dodgers. The Angels were so hapless that some of their advertising highlighted their visiting opponents: "Come out to see Mickey Mantle and the New York Yankees!"

Of course, they went on to win the World Series decades later. But in my childhood, they were a "maybe next year" team. Maybe next year they would win more games than they lost. Maybe next year they would climb up from the bottom of the standings.

We have a "maybe next year" tree by the street in front of our house. We needed a tree out there to block some of the summer sun that routinely fried our lawn. We also craved fall color, so when a landscaper showed us pictures of a maple called a "Fall Fiesta," we said, "Wow, look at all those fiery leaves! Put one in right now!"

So he did. And all the budding leaves fell off, and the tree went dormant. We looked at our bare little tree all winter, praying that dormant was something different from dead.

The tree budded in the spring. Of course, it hardly cast any shade, little thing that it was. The lawn still turned brown when summer came.

And the fall colors turned out to be less than a fiesta—some yellow, mostly brown, and then all gone.

Maybe next year?

The next year was better. The tree budded in the spring, and there was noticeable fresh growth on top. It grew taller. Its leaves seemed fuller. It didn't shield the lawn from the sun, but it cast a respectable shadow where the dog liked to pee on hot days.

There were some deep red leaves in the mix for autumn.

Maybe something more next year?

Each year adds. It grows taller; the trunk is stouter, and that tree actually shades the main part of the lawn except for a few days when the sun is impossibly high in the sky. And it totally lights up in an array of warm colors to tell us fall is here. Fiesta!

Digging Around

Like waiting on a plant to bloom, taking care of an autistic person requires patient hope. Your heart, and maybe your mind, will break if you are into precise timelines. "Next September our kids will achieve 'X'" must be held loosely. "X" might happen in October, or November, or the following spring, or September two years out, or not for a very long time.

We agonized for years about our son's inability to tell us when he was sick. He couldn't say, "I have a headache." And his dislike for sustained effort meant he wouldn't cooperate with our "process of elimination" questions. He would say "Yes" to anything just to get rid of us.

"Does your head hurt?"

"Yes."

"Does your stomach hurt?"

"Yes."

"Do cats fly on tiny, little wings?"

"Yes."

Trying to teach him to point at what hurt wasn't any better. He would wave his hand up and down his body, like Vanna White displaying the board on *Wheel of Fortune*.

But he had a recent breakthrough. He seemed a bit off, so Melissa asked him, "How do you feel?" Usually, he'll just say

"Fine" or "Happy" even if his face and tone say anything other than those qualities.

But this time, he responded to his mom with, "Do you have a stomach ache?" Yes, it was a question when we wanted a statement—but it was his way of sharing precise information with us.

Like hopelessly loyal sports fans or amateur gardeners, caregivers have to keep telling themselves, "Maybe next year." And in the next year, or tomorrow, or a few seconds from now, a once-abandoned hope arrives as a surprise.

Fertilizer

Gardeners like ourselves must learn and relearn "deferred gratification." We might want to stick a stalk in the ground and see a tree the next day, and we want to think that one or two sit-downs with an exercise book will have our kid reading literature in time for kindergarten.

But when it comes to caring for someone with special needs, it is important to hold a goal patiently. If it is a good goal (helpful and realistic to the person in our care, not a fantasy to please ourselves), it is worth holding onto in heart, mind, and habits over many seasons.

Jesus' follower Paul put it this way, "For in this hope we were saved. But hope that is seen is no hope at all. Who hopes for what they already have?" (Romans 8:24 NIV).

Like travelers using the four cardinal directions on a map, people who follow Jesus find spiritual orientation from three cardinal virtues: "faith, hope and love" (I Corinthians 13:13 NIV).

Hope keeps us looking to the horizon, to what's next. We hope for what we do not see or have, but believe what can be out there.

Hope allows us to act with purpose, believing that our efforts are worthwhile and taking us toward a good destination. It means long seasons of waiting, of doing the right stuff over and over even when a desired result isn't coming into view.

When we come to terms with hope, we find that it isn't

really about a particular event, thing, or outcome, but it's about coming face-to-face with the one who is calling us forward. It is about meeting up with Jesus and continuing the journey forward with him. Paul seems to have been a blooming idiot of sorts since he discovered this through much trial and error.

"And we know that in all things God works for the good of those who love him, who have been called according to his purpose" (Romans 8:28 NIV).

XIV. ANNUALS

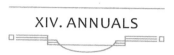

One symptom of my blooming idiocy is the fantasy that I can set stuff up, walk away, and let it take care of itself.

Serving my delusion here in South Dakota are the hardy regional shrubs sported in most planter beds. They go dormant for the winter then burst out in new life every spring. I've been saying "sleep well" and "welcome back" to ours for the last ten years. Beyond trimming them back a bit in the fall and weeding in the summer, they don't need much. The spring thaw and summer thunderstorms seem to give them plenty of water. They're just there.

But they're not all that pretty. If you want pretty, you want flowers. And if you want flowers here on the Northern Plains, only annuals will do. Annuals are flowers that grow, live, and die in the same year. No dormancy, no automatic revival next season. No set 'em up and let 'em go. You start over every year.

We did well with annuals in some of our Southern California gardens. We filled one bed with pansies of all different hues, and they lit up the white plaster exterior of the house.

But annuals are work. Like all things lovely, they can be delicate. They need protection from weeds, bugs, and varmints like romping dogs or children. The distance between too much and too little water isn't much, and a step too far in either direction is fatal.

Here in South Dakota, the weather extremes must be navigated. If you plant before spring locks in, a frost can occur, and the annuals are history. In the midst of a broiling summer, a thunderstorm can sweep in and dump inches of water. You have mud puddles where your planting once shined. The blazing sun in the bright blue sky, like the pattern for our state flag, fries fragile flowers.

The result is that we're on hiatus from planting flowers here. We tried a hanging basket on the front porch last year, but that died in a week. I stick to the trees and shrubs, who indulge my "set 'em up and let 'em go" idiocy.

Digging Around

Joey's autism does yeoman work of blowing up my fantasy of predictable order. Just when something seems to work, it breaks down.

For example, Joey loved the water. One of my first memories of him appearing "normal" in public was at a beach where he ran out to the water and let the waves chase him back, all the while laughing just like the other little kids.

All of us are native Californians, but Joey's the only one ever to go out on a surfboard, shivering, and grinning all at once, thanks to a special day camp for kids with autism put on by a pro surfer.

But it wasn't just the ocean. Any water made caring for Joey easier. The best way to soothe him was to get him back to the beach, into a pool, or, even better, a hot tub.

Then he stopped liking water. We signed him up and paid the fee for pool access with one of his summer programs. And he just stopped going into the water. He lost all interest with no rhyme or reason.

And then there were haircuts. He has a great young lady who cuts his hair. We've been with her for several years. He goes in, sits compliantly in her chair, responds to her commands to "look up" or "turn your head," and makes it easy on us all.

That changed last week when he wouldn't get out of the waiting area when it was time to sit in the stylist's chair. I couldn't coax him. The stylist, sweet as can be, couldn't convince him. He just smiled and crossed his arms over his chest in charming defiance. I tried to move him, but he resisted. Then he got up, went to the barber's chair, and shoved it off of its rubber floor mat and into the wall. The stylist finally offered to come cut his hair in the waiting area, and he consented to that.

Autism is known for "repetitive behaviors." But sometimes the only constant seems to be change. Caregivers don't get to "set it up and let it go" any more than gardeners can depend upon flowers on the Northern Plains.

Fertilizer

Religion is one way that people try to bring some comfortable order to life. We look for God or some representative of God, like a church or moral code, to be steady and predictable. We want a god we can wind up and let go, kind of an annual who shows up at the right time but isn't too dramatic and certainly doesn't ask much of us.

Jesus identified this "wind it up and let it go" mentality with an example from do-it-yourself construction.

> As for everyone who comes to me and hears my words and puts them into practice, I will show you what they are like. They are like a man building a house, who dug down deep and laid the foundation on rock. When a flood came, the torrent struck that house but could not shake it, because it was well built. But the one who hears my words and does not put them into practice is like a man who built a house on the ground without a foundation. The moment the torrent struck that house, it collapsed and its destruction was complete.
> (Luke 6:47-49 NIV)

His words about building a well-anchored house sound like "set it up and let it go." English puts his words in the past tense, but in the Greek of the New Testament, he's talking about continually building and constantly doing. You know, like caregiving or keeping delicate flowers alive.

What are his ultimate words for us to "be doing"?

Jesus said, "A new command I give you: Love one another. As I have loved you, so you must love one another" (John 13:34 NIV).

His love is constant, weathering all the twists and turns of our lives and patiently guiding us to grow and change. And his love isn't something we just wind up and let go; it is something to which he calls us as active and constant participants. As he always loves us, we are to grow in our capacity to love one another.

"Wind it up and let it go" implies keeping something or someone—a garden, another person, Jesus—at a distance. But Jesus tells us to go all in, with every aspect of who we are. "'The most important one,' answered Jesus, 'is this: 'Hear, O Israel: The Lord our God, the Lord is one. Love the Lord your God with all your heart and with all your soul and with all your mind and with all your strength.' The second is this: 'Love your neighbor as yourself.' There is no commandment greater than these'" (Mark 12:29-31 NIV).

Loving isn't predictably seasonal like my shrubs. You don't "fall in love" once and then it takes care of itself. You nurture it and work at it, like with more fragile annual flowers. It will wither without attention. Too much emotion will drown it, too little will dry it up. Dwelling on our own failures and frustrations can keep us from kneeling down to the messy work of loving those in our care.

Love teaches us to see others as God's beloved people, no matter how much of an unholy terror they might be from time to time. To "be doing" the love that Jesus describes is our strength in the face of all the changes and challenges. Love is the only possible permanence we can find. Jesus says that it is our strength here and now, and our promise of eternity. "[Love] always protects, always trusts, always hopes, always perseveres. Love never fails. But where there are prophecies, they will cease; where there are tongues, they will be stilled; where there is knowledge, it will pass away" (1 Corinthians 13:7-8 NIV).

If I might offer a blooming idiot's paraphrase, "Love does not wind up and let go. It stays connected, come what may."

XV. IT SMELLS GOOD WHEN YOU TRY
AND TRY AGAIN

Gardenias are one of Melissa's favorite flowers. Their hypnotic perfume is one of the pleasures of gardening.

The first house we bought together had a row of gardenia shrubs along the front walkway, which had been planted by the previous owners. Melissa was hooked the first time they flowered. Wherever we went in years to come, she decided we would always plant gardenias. But the lofty intention produced a low yield.

At our next place, Melissa tried and tried. She could never find the right spot for ideal sunlight or figure out the proper watering for the fragile beauties. We gave up on gardenias at that house.

Two houses later, in a cooler setting near the coast, Melissa decided to try again. She went to a local nursery, determined to get all the supplies and, most of all, information to make gardenias grow.

She later told me she had cornered a nursery employee. "I wasn't going to let her go until I had all the information I needed," she said. "I hit her with every possible question. Do they go in the ground or pots? Special soil, fertilizer or both? Tell me the precise sun, water, and feeding instructions. Do I move them around? Do I talk to them? Kiss them?"

It was an informative visit and lucrative for the nursery. Melissa came home with large, terra-cotta pots and bags of special soil that gardenias were said to fancy, and, of course, the honored guests: the small gardenia shrubs themselves.

The pots were set up in a spot that caught morning sun and provided afternoon shade: plenty of light but not too much heat. In went the dirt, I mean, potting soil. The plants were lifted from their temporary plastic launch pads and landed in their new terra-cotta worlds, followed by carefully measured helpings of water.

Success. The gardenias thrived at that house under Melissa's care. It was the result of sustained effort through seasons of disappointment.

That garden became our most fragrant. The gardenias perfumed one end while star jasmine climbed a fence at the other. Our noses feasted day and night.

Digging Around

Some flowers are so sensitive that even sincere efforts to nurture them fail. Caregiving is an exercise in worthwhile efforts that, for long stretches, don't seem to be working.

Joey is in his twenties now. For two decades, we've struggled to help him use words. "Use your words" was one of the prompts that echoed around our family for years. It was a prolonged attempt to help him replace noises, gestures, and even violence with simple phrases.

Suddenly, he's talking up a storm. He's using complete sentences to indicate what he needs. The folks at his day program are telling us that he's actually conversing instead of parroting movie lines and song lyrics.

We had quite the conversation at home last night. Joey was using a repetitive phrase with Melissa. It's based on a nickname he developed for friends of ours from years ago. The wife would tell their kids, "Time for beddy-bye," and he decided that her name was "Wedgy-Pie." Their place became known as "Wedgy-Pie's house."

They had one of the animated Charlie Brown movies, and Joey always tried to sneak off with it. They would catch him in the act and take it back. So Joey developed his own simple retelling of that event, in which he says "What did Wedgy-Pie do?" And we are expected to answer, "Wedgy-Pie took the

Charlie Brown movie."

But last night, Melissa made eye contact with him and said, "Wedgy-Pie was what Gregg and Annie said at their house. Gregg and Annie had the Charlie Brown movie."

Joey processed this, came to me in a different room and said, "The Charlie Brown movie was at Gregg and Annie's house. Gregg and Annie took the Charlie Brown movie."

Now this sounds like a trivial little tale, but it was a major breakthrough. Joey absorbed and shared a story, not just a phrase he memorized. He received new information, reinterpreted a memory, and then sought to communicate it to a third party.

I know. I know. That's no big deal. That's what humans do.

But it wasn't what Joey did. For twenty years. And last night, long seasons of much trial and much error gave way to growth. That evening, our home had a sweet smell, not of gardenias, but of success.

So much of caregiving is just sticking with it and enduring trial and error. Lots of error. Over the years, Melissa potted many gardenias that never grew. Then one day she asked that home and garden store employee about it, got a bit of good advice about sunshine, and set the pots in the right place to catch just enough sun but not too much.

Melissa tried something new with Joey that night when she coached him to take in, process and share information instead of echo sounds. He bloomed, too.

Fertilizer

It isn't easy to tell when to stick with something, as Melissa did with gardenias and our family did with Joey's language, and when to call something fruitless and give up.

Jesus warned his followers that their path would be long and difficult, but ultimately it would result in joy beyond description. Jesus said, "Very truly I tell you, you will weep and mourn while the world rejoices. You will grieve, but your grief will turn to joy. A woman giving birth to a child has pain because her time has come; but when her baby is born she forgets the anguish because of her joy that a child is born into the world" (John 16:20-21 NIV).

Jesus is teaching about eternal matters: the hard path from this life to heavenly life. But along the way we are prepared by numerous "dress rehearsals," in which long seasons of struggle are replaced by great joy.

We need to take and cuddle these breakthrough moments as if holding newborn babies. They are signs of a loving God who "...is not unjust; he will not forget your work and the love you have shown him as you have helped his people and continue to help them" (Hebrews 6:10 NIV).

Remember, Jesus is the master gardener who says, "Give it another season." Melissa found that years of empty gardenia pots could give way to glorious plants that perfumed her whole garden. She helped Joey discover a sentence to replace years of baby talk.

Our loving efforts, even ones that seem fruitless, can be part of a new, beautiful, and fragrant season that Jesus is creating through us.

XVI. SCRUFFY FRIENDS

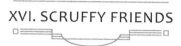

I've mentioned that we have hardy bushes that are the opposite of fragile annual flowers. They sit in the planter beds on both sides of our front walkway.

We have some affection for them. I trim them back when they turn brown in the fall, wishing them a good rest through their winter dormancy. And I rejoice when they bloom again in the spring. I find myself saying to them, "Welcome back! Happy Easter!"

Melissa adopted one in particular. It's one of the most visible, sitting right at the head of the walkway. If it isn't trimmed, it poofs up with broad leaves and round, heavy flowers that make it sag until it looks like it's wilting. Melissa made it a fall tradition to cut it back to a tight ball of twigs, and it blooms better under her personal care.

I even grieved over the few of these plants we lost one year. We had "ice dams" when a short thaw gave way to an abrupt freeze and solidified the water in the rain gutters. This can cause water to back up into the walls of the house, so we had a crew come over to melt the blockage with some chemicals. But the chemicals dripped down and killed a couple of plants closest to the house. It gave me some heartache when they didn't come back to life in the spring.

It's weird to have these plants tug at our hearts. They aren't all that pretty. Some are just tufts of tall wild grass. Others are thorny and muted in their colors. Sometimes after trimming them, their spring bloom looks kind of lumpy. Some of them are just scruffy by nature.

But they mark our seasons, especially the end of the long winter. They belong with the songbirds that come back every spring, or the "snow birds"—friends who winter in warmer states and return to us smiling and tan.

Digging Around

We wouldn't go out looking for scruffy bushes, but the ones in our yard have our affection because they are part of our home. We see the loveliness of what we nurture. I suppose that's a reason all parents see the beauty in their own kids.

Joey has his attractive features: hazel eyes that light up when he wears green, his tall and slender build, and his radiant smile. He looked downright elegant in a suit and tie with one long leg crossed over the other, perched on a chair at his brother's wedding.

Then again, I can show plenty of pictures where he looks just plain weird. His eyes angle off in the wrong direction from what he's doing. He manages to have bed head no matter how much attention we put into his hair. He gets his clothes all disarrayed and won't straighten them out. He contorts his arms, fingers, and face like he's lost control of nerves and muscles.

The scruffiness is beyond looks. There are the messes he makes in our home. There are the intrusions of noise and emotional upsets in quiet nights. There are the lost opportunities to travel or even spend a day with friends because it is beyond his physical or behavioral limits.

But we love him. He's part of us in his handsome moments and in the cartoonish goofiness of his autism. Our lives—our hearts—would be diminished without our scruffy seasons of Joey.

Fertilizer

One of the stronger criticisms that atheists level at believers is, "Your God is just an escape, a fantasy you project to help you avoid the hard facts of life."

But Christians follow Jesus, who shows us that God loves

the scruffy world so much that he makes himself scruffy to help us. As one of the ancient prophets said in a verse that points to Jesus: "He grew up before him like a tender shoot, and like a root out of dry ground. He had no beauty or majesty to attract us to him, nothing in his appearance that we should desire him" (Isaiah 53:2 NIV).

The faith, hope, and love that sustain us are not in a Prince Charming or another pleasant fantasy. Yes, Christians confess that Jesus is perfect, and he lived in complete obedience to the will of God. But to accomplish this Jesus got down in the dirt with us and did his work in weakness and vulnerability. As Paul writes in the New Testament, "[Jesus], who, being in very nature God, did not consider equality with God something to be used to his own advantage; rather, he made himself nothing by taking the very nature of a servant, being made in human likeness. And being found in appearance as a man, he humbled himself by becoming obedient to death—even death on a cross!" (Philippians 2:6-8 NIV).

We can look right at what the world sees as humiliation and defeat and discover unmatched victory over evil and death. Christians are not perfect, but season after season our scruffy lives grow because Jesus loves and tends us through life's hard realities.

It is this perspective that helps Melissa and me. Jesus is not an escape from taking care of Joey, but the one who encourages us to stay in the scruffiness. Jesus can transform caregiving from a grim duty into a precious, beautiful, and holy offering to God.

Sincere Christian faith endures sufferings and setbacks and keeps following Jesus. He looks past our flaws and failures with eyes of love, because he sees his coming kingdom as more complete and beautiful with us in it. Where human eyes see only scruffiness, the eyes of faith see beauty.

XVII. THEY ARE WHAT THEY EAT?

Before Melissa and I met, before there was a Joey, I worked in San Pedro, the harbor area of Los Angeles. There was a man I used to drop in on, who spent most of his time at home because of a chronic illness. He was an Englishman, properly discreet about a big secret. On days when he felt up to it, he and his wife would take me out to their backyard for tea. They had a true English garden. There were perfect rows of hedges and colorful flowers. It looked like an illustration from a Beatrix Potter story.

One day, I asked him how he kept it up, given his illness.

"Well, the wife does much of the work," he replied, "but I add a special fertilizer." He left it hanging. He didn't reveal the secret.

Rude Yank that I am, I pushed on. "Which is?"

"Fish parts." His eyes twinkled. "Heads, guts, the lot. I drive down to the docks when the boats come in, and they give me the parts they'd be tossing."

I'd been out on some of the charter boats, on which the crew filleted the patrons' catch. I always paid for that service rather than deal with the gross parts they toss. But that man's vibrant English garden didn't lie; the disgusting remains produced great beauty.

I confess that in all my years of trying to grow stuff, I never dabbled in his method. I guess I preferred to be a blooming idiot rather than a stinking success.

Digging Around

If you're raising someone with autism, you've heard about diet. It is a fact that diet contributes to some autistic kids' progress in social and academic skills. There are anecdotal cases of kids moving from special education to mainstream classes after a diet adjustment. There's lurking hope for that one magical menu that will "cure" autism.

"Gluten free" is one of the most highly recommended. Joey had a great home therapist who was 100 percent certain that there would be progress if Joey would go gluten free.

"But he loves pizza," we warned.

"They have gluten free crusts now. Oh, and no more white buns or mustard on his cheeseburgers."

Melissa was ready to rebel right then and there. It was not easy to get Joey to eat, and now we were being told to eliminate everything he liked, down to the last drop of mustard.

But we gave it a try. There was a market that specialized in all the gluten free, healthy fare. It was a bit of a drive, but I loaded up.

Joey gave it a try, too. And he hated it. He wanted no part of the faux pizza that replaced greasy, cheesy goodness. He wanted both ketchup *and* mustard on his burgers and a nutrition-free white bun that was just flour and air, not some dry, healthy thing that was closer to a parakeet's seed block.

In fact, his behavior deteriorated. Instead of effort interspersed with pleasures, his days became all work, all the time. His anxiety and temper went up, and he resisted activities that had been agreeable before. He cried. He pushed food away.

We endured the therapist's dour expression as we went back to the gross stuff Joey loved. Sure enough, Joey became happier and more cooperative, as if we'd found that magic menu for autism in the not-so-healthy foods that "normal" kids like. Like a gorgeous garden nourished on fish heads, Joey's happiness blossomed with some salty, carb-heavy pleasures at the dinner table.

Fertilizer

Food and faith come together quite a bit. Sure, church people get together for shared meals called pot lucks or covered dish suppers or something else depending upon where we live. Prayer groups meet in coffee shops (hipster prayer groups in coffee houses); churchmen hold chili cook-off contests, etc.

But Jesus left a particular meal for his followers, above and apart from any other food they might share.

> For I received from the Lord what I also passed on to you: The Lord Jesus, on the night he was betrayed, took bread, and when he had given thanks, he broke it and said, "This is my body, which is for you; do this in remembrance of me." In the same way, after supper he took the cup, saying, "This cup is the new covenant in my blood; do this, whenever you drink it, in remembrance of me." For whenever you eat this bread and drink this cup, you proclaim the Lord's death until he comes.
> (1 Corinthians 11:23-26 NIV)

How weird that Jesus tells his followers to gather and eat what sounds to be blunt and gross. In churches where kids receive Holy Communion, you can hear the whiny objections, "We're gonna drink blood?" and then see the sour little faces when they taste wine for the first time, suggesting that blood might have been better after all.

But the point is that we are not worshiping a distant "maybe he's there, maybe he's not" god. We are uniting with the God, who chose to unite with us, even to share the gross sufferings of body, heart and mind that go with being human.

We "proclaim his death" not just with words, but in this meal. His broken body and spilled blood are what the world chose "to toss," like fish heads, but which we know will give us life just as sure as fish heads grew my friend's glorious garden.

And like Joey, we come for the gross meal that comforts us rather than all the stuff the world tells us is "healthy." We come to the table and put out our hands, all equally empty and in need, rather than compare who has the most, or does the most, or gives the most, or who excels in any of what the world deems "good."

We put ourselves in the care of the only one who is good, and who put himself into the gross, flesh-and-blood realities of our human life. The fellow with the English garden seemed eccentric to go begging for "the head, the guts, the lot they toss out," but his hillside flourished. Melissa and I might have been labeled lazy or "bad parents" when we ordered oily pizza instead of vegan burgers for Joey, but we reached for what helped him most.

The world pressures and tempts us all to grasp at what's prettiest, well packaged and correct "on paper." We reach instead for Jesus, who died an ugly death on a cross to give us new life... "we preach Christ crucified ... the power of God and the wisdom of God. For the foolishness of God is wiser than human wisdom, and the weakness of God is stronger than human strength" (1 Corinthians 1:23-25 NIV).

XVIII. SOLE SURVIVOR

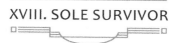

A small green plant sits on our kitchen table. Long, leafy tendrils coil out and try to wrap around the closest chair. It doesn't require much care. All I have to do is give it a splash of water once a week and pull off an occasional brown leaf. I turn the basket once a month because the plant gets lopsided, leaning toward the sliding glass door where the morning sun shines. It's like reminding a kid to stop slouching and keep good posture.

What's remarkable is that Melissa and I haven't managed to neglect this dude unto death. It's been there on the kitchen table for years. It was a gift from some coworkers. We were struggling financially, and I took a second job parking cars at a medical center. When my mom died, the other valets sent the plant as a sympathy gift. Given our record with indoor plants, I wondered which would come first, mom's scheduled funeral or the plant's consignment to the trash can.

But the plant's still there, green, grabbing onto chair backs and lolling like a cat in the morning sun. It doesn't flower; it's not pretty or shapely. But it delights me. Because it lives.

Digging Around

It doesn't take much to keep that plant going. Likewise, a little care for the caregiver goes a long way.

I was driving home from work one nasty winter day, grumbling to myself about all the domestic effort that lay ahead. Lo and behold, one of the neighbors had cleared the snow from my driveway and sidewalk. I swear it felt like finding a letter with a million dollars from some long-lost relative. That simple kindness transformed my attitude toward the rest of the day.

The demands of raising and caring for a person with autism can produce pity parties. Words like "unfair," "overwhelmed" and "inadequate" pepper a caregiver's speech. However, the other side of that is how small blessings loom larger.

Melissa and I try to share the tasks created by Joey's needs. Needless to say, some days one of us gets stuck with more of the effort than the other. Speaking for myself, the bits of time gained when Melissa spares me a chore or two feel like vacations. A half-hour here, fifteen minutes there, and the pace of life is so much better.

And it is hard to describe the joy we experience when we hear the blessed words, "Hey, I'll watch Joey for you while you (fill in some desired activity other than caregiving)."

That plant on our kitchen table sprawls out as a sign. It reminds us of my coworkers' compassion, but it also reminds us of ourselves. Like us, just a bit of care keeps it alive and reaching toward the light.

Fertilizer

Melissa and I gave up on indoor plants because of our many failures to keep them alive. So just imagine how caregiving challenges our joy. It generates so much hurt and defeat.

Pity parties are a twisted way to feel better. But God didn't create us for gloom-fests. A Christian sitting in prison wrote:

Rejoice in the Lord always. I will say it again: Rejoice! Let your gentleness be evident to all. The Lord is near. Do not be anxious about anything, but in every situation, by prayer and petition, with thanksgiving, present your requests to God. And the peace of God, which transcends all understanding, will guard your hearts and your minds in Christ Jesus (Philippians 4:4-7 NIV).

Our nature, the true desire of our heart, is to rejoice in the goodness of God. It can take some work to let this kind of joy grow. We have to dig out bits of gratitude in the simple moments and events of our days. Our active part is to be prayerfully aware "in everything." We are challenged to dwell, by faith, on the assumption that God loves us and is working to bring us a peace "which transcends all understanding."

Rejoicing and giving thanks are "God's will for us." Hear that properly. Not, "God's will is that you smile and say thank you, so suck it up and do what he says." Rather, God wants you to have a glad and grateful heart and sends Christ Jesus into the midst of your challenges to "guard your heart and mind" and set you free to discover joy.

Start small. Savor the small gestures offered by others. Delight in short breaks from heavy lifting. Giggle because one low maintenance house plant is a survivor, in spite of your blooming idiocy.

Somewhere in those little spiritual delights, you'll connect with Jesus, who is their source. Lean toward him in prayer, like my plant toward the sunshine.

XIX. TALK DIRTY

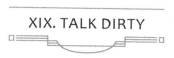

We were the owners of a brand-new house. The yard was clay, completely unready to support green life. It needed to become "earth" before we could plant grass, let alone flowers, bushes, and trees.

The landscaper came in with machinery that roughed up the clay and then layered in lots of soil. Yes, we paid to import dirt to our new little kingdom.

The transformation was dramatic. The expanses of hard, hot, crusty clay gave way to swatches of rich, dark earth that looked like coffee grounds. Once the dirt was down, grass seeds were shot into it with bursts of water, and we had proper suburban green all around our home.

Later we started planting trees. Wielding a shovel and a post-hole contraption, I got down through the nice soil and into that clay. It threw the tools back at me. I counterattacked. It was backbreaking work. Finally, holes appeared and were refilled with good planting soil that would welcome young tree roots.

Such are the wonders of blooming idiocy, in which dirt makes a difference.

Digging Around

Joey's autism diagnosis came when he was about two years old. Melissa remembers the news as "a cold, hard thing." That moment in the pediatrician's office was vacant and lifeless, like the clay moonscape when we first arrived at that new house.

Just as we called in contractors to spread good dirt and

get our yard started, we found ourselves calling in experts of all kinds to nurture Joey's life: Pediatric psychiatrists, audiologists (to rule out hearing loss as his reason for ignoring us), neurologists (to monitor his brain for seizure activity), and later, physical and occupational therapists of various kinds. And with all the experts, there was the day-to-day labor put in by Joey's resident amateurs: Melissa and me.

Like breaking through the clay, the work was hard. Progress did not come easily, but it came. None of our yards became horticultural award-winners. And Joey was not "cured" of autism. But life came forth—green life in the yards and a sweet humanity in Joey. He showed himself to be good soil for growth. Not everything we planted in his life took root, but so much did.

Fertilizer

Being amateurs and idiots, we need help to bring out good fruit in the lives of those in our care. God sends his Word, full of life. Jesus looks to see if we are the type of "dirt" that can receive it.

> This is the meaning of the parable: The seed is the word of God. Those along the path are the ones who hear, and then the devil comes and takes away the word from their hearts, so that they may not believe and be saved. Those on the rocky ground are the ones who receive the word with joy when they hear it, but they have no root. They believe for a while, but in the time of testing they fall away. The seed that fell among thorns stands for those who hear, but as they go on their way they are choked by life's worries, riches and pleasures, and they do not mature. But the seed on good soil stands for those with a noble and good heart, who hear the word, retain it, and by persevering produce a crop.
> (Luke 8:11-15 NIV)

Remember, we couldn't punch grass seed into clay. We needed to have good soil for the lawns to grow. What kind of "ground" are you? Can the seed, the Word of God, get in to bring the help you need?

Jesus tells us about four kinds of dirt. There's the "path," pounded so solid that the seed just can't get in. Are you hardened in some way that needs softening?

Then there's rocky ground. The seed can get in, but it's hard for the roots to spread out and grow. The plant can't survive harsh conditions when they come. Is your faith superficial? Can you let God's word go deeper, down into the depths of your heart, so that it brings life even in the midst of hardship?

The third one is the weed patch. I'll bet that many of us who care for people with autism are weed patches. We have so many cares, we worry about resources, and we feel pleasure-deprived much of the time. Can we pluck out some of our weeds and make space for the Word of God to grow in their place?

We must pray and work to be the fourth kind: the good soil. We need to be folks who "hold God's word in honest and good hearts, and bear fruit with patience." When Melissa and I have been dirt like that, it's made all the difference, for Joey and us. Because God's word teaches us to forgive as we are forgiven, we've been able to embrace Joey in calming love even when he's hurt us during violent meltdowns. He has a loving home, and we delight in sharing life with him because God's Word tells us about sacrifice as a defining quality of true love. It's God's Word that tells us how steady faithfulness means more than rapid results or having everything our own way. It is Jesus' way that helps us "bear fruit" together.

XX. ROCKY ROAD

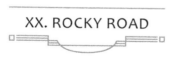

We've tried to protect various planter beds from weeds. It's a big effort that, in our experience, yields only short-lived success.

First, you must strip everything off the surface: rocks, dead plants, existing weeds, everything down to the dirt. You rake or otherwise soften up the dirt and then try to lay down these sheets of material that are supposed to let the water and fertilizer pass down into the soil while keeping out weeds. Then you exhaust yourself lugging heavy bags or wheelbarrows full of some natural-looking cover. After all, you don't want your flower beds to look like overgrown garbage bags. So you lay down rocks, redwood chips, or something scenic.

Oh, wait! Did I mention that before you do that, you need to cut spots in the fabric where you'll be putting in the flowers and shrubs? I didn't? Well, then, remove some of that rock you just hauled in and make the cuts. Oh, and don't worry. I'm sure the weeds will never think to sneak in where you perforated the weed-preventing material.

So, get it all done in the spring, and you'll have weeks of garden beauty. The little flowering plants that you put in the holes will bloom and light up your yard. And by the end of summer, you'll notice other little plants joining them from places where the rocks or your own incisions have pierced the sheets you laid.

Yep. Weeds. Dig it all up, and do it again. Or just surrender to the reality that you'll be pulling weeds just as much as before you did all the backbreaking work.

Digging Around

The weeds grow outside. Inside the house, mornings go something like this: the dog's snout nudges me awake before sunrise. I shave and then let the dog out for her morning business. I come in and turn on the awesome coffee maker that Melissa got me, and the bean-grinding roar gets Joey stirring. I hear Joey thumping around down the hall, and my peripheral vision catches the glow of his bathroom light. If I'm lucky, the coffee is brewed, and I've downed some. If not, I just stumble down the hall to Joey first.

He's twenty years old. This exact morning routine has been playing out for, well, at least, the ten years we've had the dog. I get to Joey's bathroom, and the routine continues. No matter how many times we've been through this, he needs help combing his hair into anything other than bed head. His shirt is likely half tucked in. The waistband of his boxers shows from some angle. And his pants are on backward a good percentage of the time.

"Joey, the tag goes ...?"

"The tag goes in the back."

But he never uses that information to orient his pants before stepping into them. So I help him get them on right.

At least we've escaped the fashion disasters of his earlier years. The clothes we buy are all simple primary colors, interchangeable tops and bottoms, so he can't mix stripes and plaids or anything like that anymore. But it's been a decade of this, morning in and morning out. And I'm weary, coffee or no coffee.

No amount of work eliminates all the weeds; no amount of work overcomes autism.

Fertilizer

I forgot to mention part of my morning routine, something that predates Joey, the dog, and even my coffee guzzling. It's morning prayer, which I dive into even before the coffee brews.

I spend time reading the Bible, in particular, the Psalms,

which are God-given prayers that pour out the full range of human emotion. Whatever is filling our heads and tugging our hearts, the Psalms have a way of bringing it to God for help.

That first-thing-in-the-morning prayer time has been the anchor of my life. It has been a time of inspiration and gratitude in good seasons, a refuge and comfort in bad stretches, and good counsel when I've been confused. It takes all of the temporary things of life and puts them in perspective, laying them out in the presence of the eternal God.

It's like those "You are here" dots on the map of a shopping mall, a college, a medical center, or another large campus. Our agenda might have us feeling like the weight of the world is on our shoulders, but we are just one dot in a big venue full of dots, feeling just as much pressure. Jesus knows that, and says, "Come to me, all you who are weary and burdened, and I will give you rest. Take my yoke upon you and learn from me, for I am gentle and humble in heart, and you will find rest for your souls. For my yoke is easy and my burden is light" (Matthew 11:28-30 NIV).

Jesus says, "Spend time with me, and I'll show you how to carry stuff. And it won't be nearly as heavy a load as the one you've planted in your head."

XXI. FORGET ME NOT

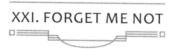

Blooming idiot that I am, I still know there's an actual flower called a Forget-Me-Not. This is not about that. It's about an envelope in my desk at work. It's one of those little seed packets they have on racks near the supermarket checkout stands. You know, the "impulse buy" products.

"Gee, it's almost lunchtime, so instead of rushing home to cook these vegetables in my cart, I think I'll just grab this candy bar to eat in the car."

"Wow, that *Cosmopolitan* magazine says I can look like their cover model and have a great love life. Better buy that, since it's right here at the checkout stand."

"Why, look here. A whole rack of flower and vegetable seeds. You know, I've always daydreamed about being a farmer."

I'm proud to say I didn't get the seed packet in my office as an impulse buy. It was a gift from Melissa's longtime friend, Pat. She gave it to me when I started a new job as a reminder that great achievements start out tiny. A sign to remember (forget not) the possibilities when challenges or setbacks arrived.

So it's never been opened. It just travels with me, a forget-me-not sign of a caring friend and an important message.

Digging Around

There are good plants and bad ones, and there's a poisonous seed sometimes planted in the minds of caregivers: "That condition must be the result of bad parenting." In fact, one early categorization of autism was "Cold Mothering Syndrome" or some Freudian freak-out like that. As one mother of a child with autism lamented in a Facebook chat, "Moms always feel guilty about any 'flaws' in our kids, whether it is rational or not. Moms are just like that."

Over the years, Joey's autism has remained "profound." He's never going to do traditional schoolwork and will need support and direction to keep up on basic life skills and any kind of employment efforts. There's plenty of room for Mom and Dad, to feel like withered failures.

But one of the ways in which our blooming idiocy blesses our son's life is his mom's constant affection for him. She's always maintained a high level of touch, chatter, singing and emotion for him. (Notice that this didn't "cure" his autism. So the flip side is that the absence of it wouldn't have "caused" the disorder. So be gentle with yourselves, moms.) He's twenty years old, and she still tucks him in at night, offering a little prayer, making sure that a comforting weighted blanket covers him and always getting his biggest smile for her effort.

This isn't just feel-good stuff; it is life-giving. We've had medical, educational, and therapeutic professionals remark on Joey's emotional connection to the world around him. He laughs at funny things, shows empathy (OK, not the full load but certainly a good measure), and is anxious when a member of the family is missing. He could hardly eat his breakfast one morning because the dog, which he usually ignores, was at the groomer. "Lily's not here?" was his refrain, accompanied by his knotted brow and frown.

In all of our blooming idiocy, running after different "techniques" and resources to give Joey a good life, some basic affection has been our most fruitful contribution.

In the midst of the big dramatic interventions that caregiving requires, don't forget the seemingly small things from which life springs—those "mustard seeds" that seem puny but are poised to grow and shelter the lives of those in our care. Pat's gift still encourages me many years later. Melissa's voice and touch are in Joey's heart and are part of this happy young man he's grown to be.

Fertilizer

That little seed packet in my office holds mustard seeds. Our friend Pat understood something Jesus said, so when she gave me the present, she didn't have to say anything. The twinkle in her eye carried the divine message: "Again [Jesus] said, 'What shall we say the kingdom of God is like, or what parable shall we use to describe it? It is like a mustard seed, which is the smallest of all seeds on earth. Yet when planted, it grows and becomes the largest of all garden plants, with such big branches that the birds can perch in its shade'" (Mark 4:30-32 NIV).

The kingdom of God, Jesus tells us, starts out in little, common things. There's nothing impressive or exotic about mustard seeds. Some would say they're just the start of another weed. Yet they grow up bushy and provide shelter to birds and seasoning to our tables.

Do not despise your lack of "expertise" when it comes to raising your autistic child. Don't despair because you feel small in the face of a tall order. If there were a perfect way to do the job, there would be a book with step-by-step directions, and we would all be following it.

But we know there's no such book. And so the greatest earthly resource to your autistic child is you. Your presence, your caring, your straining, agonizing, your hit-and-miss efforts, your love. From small stirrings in your heart, God can bring forth abundant blessings.

XXII. OUT OF CONTROL

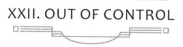

David Masumoto is a professional farmer and accomplished writer. I clipped part of a piece he wrote for the Los Angeles *Times* years before I became a blooming idiot.

"When the first storm came," he wrote. "I thought of praying, begging and pleading for the rain to stop. Another thought occurred: had I committed an evil act, a sin, and was I now being punished?

"But a part of me foolishly believed I could control nature. Allied with technology, who needed prayers? Science could do anything. If there was something wrong with my vines or grapes, I'd just spray something on to fix them."

He chronicled some of his crop disasters to bring home the lesson that nature is never 100 percent under our control. There's nothing like working the land, even a little pot in an apartment or a small plot in a suburban yard, to let you know you're not the center of the universe.

The house we rented in one town had a bed of groundcover shrubs out front. Or, at least, it did when we arrived. A gopher wiped it out, munching the plants from below. He evaded our traps and poison, and then he had a chunk of our security deposit for dessert.

Moving to South Dakota, we experienced a lawn bedeviled by the radically shifting seasonal conditions. After the spring thaw, most of the lawn would come back in lovely green, but there were always spots of barren earth. "Winter kill," the locals called it with a shrug.

So I'd scratch the dirt, toss in grass seed, water and get

it patched, only to have some other section fried to a crispy golden brown by the late summer sun.

Try as I might, I could never get the lawn to look like the green carpet of perfection maintained by a retired couple down the street. But then I didn't wrestle with nature like those two; they would be out tending it when I left for work in the morning and were still out there when I got home.

But even they suffered the irresistible natural forces. A small patch of grass, no bigger than a fist, turned brown. They blamed our dog. "Is your dog a female? They make that happen when they pee." Might have been her, maybe not. We're not in control of these things.

Digging Around

We are not against man-made interventions into what nature gave Joey. We've employed a variety of medications to control a variety of conditions. Attention span, sleep, aggression, seizures, aggression (and did I mention aggression?) were the major problem areas, and medications helped deal with all of them.

In the last year, the psychiatrist recommended he ease off several pills. We heard this with great fear and trembling. We had flashbacks to the days when it seemed that Joey would never sleep or years when punching, biting, or throwing things at us were his ways of dealing with frustration.

But the doctor prevailed. He was conscious of the potential side effects of the meds over time, and also suggested that "some conditions change with age." In other words, he was hoping that Joey might be in a better place through natural forces beyond our control.

And he was right. The removal of the attention span stimulant decreased Joey's anxiety, and a more playful, humorous side of his personality reasserted itself. Removing the sleep med caused no problems. Joey continued to sleep through the night.

The phrase "out of our control" is usually used as a negative. But Joey has taught us that some things out of our control are positives. Improvements or even "healing" of some conditions came without us having to do a thing. Yes, there are problems that we can't control, but there are also blessings that come without us lifting a finger.

Fertilizer

It's not easy to be happy when things are not as we want them to be. Lousy moods accompany lousy weather. Crummy crops and caregiving catastrophes spawn sour attitudes.

Followers of Jesus seek to break free of our tendency to tie happiness to circumstances. As the New Testament puts it, "Rejoice always, pray continually, give thanks in all circumstances; for this is God's will for you in Christ Jesus" (I Thessalonians 5:16-18 NIV).

In all circumstances? Really? That's a big problem for my mouth because it's both hard to swallow and hard to say.

It rests on the assumption that there is a plan in place, a "will of God" for our lives and that his will is for our good. This plan is out of our control and, more upsetting, it's out of our understanding much of the time. But it is "in Christ Jesus," who walked our human path of vulnerability and suffered the same afflictions that we endure. It's more that God knows us than that we know him.

Hard to swallow, hard to say. But one of the ancient prophets expressed it pretty well:

> Though the fig tree does not bud and there are no grapes on the vines, though the olive crop fails and the fields produce no food, though there are no sheep in the pen and no cattle in the stalls, yet I will rejoice in the LORD, I will be joyful in God my Savior. The Sovereign LORD is my strength; he makes my feet like the feet of a deer, he enables me to tread on the heights. For the director of music. On my stringed instruments. (Habakkuk 3:17-19 NIV)

He learned to liberate his happiness from his circumstances. Sounds like a fellow blooming idiot, doesn't he?

XXIII. FIRE ANTS!

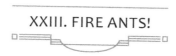

Heading out to work one sunny Southern California morning, I noticed a lump of dirt in our small front yard. "Gophers," grumbled my memory, having seen a bunch of plants devoured by the rodents at our last house.

So on the way home, I picked up poison at the hardware store. I grabbed a spade from my garage and went out to shovel the toxin into their underground construction site.

As soon as the spade poked the dirt, there was movement. I blinked, and in an instant, I dropped the tool, which was covered with rust-colored motion. Tiny ants were storming out of the mound.

I remembered something on the news about "imported Argentine fire ants." I looked up "Vector Control" for our county and phoned in. The guy who answered heard my description of the scene and said, "Yep. You got fire ants."

Well, I wasn't about to have these dinky pests dig up my lawn and possibly have me as a picnic dish. So I asked the Vector Control guy for a plan.

He said they had to have physical evidence that it was fire ants, and it was my job to get it. Step one was to get some potato chips, but not the reduced fat kind. The ants don't like those.

I happened to have some Doritos around. The fatty kind. So far, so good. I was instructed to spread them around the mound and come back later.

I obeyed, and when I returned, the chips were covered with ants. Then it was time for high-tech equipment.

"Get a Q-tip, and dip it in some liquid dish detergent. Then go up to a chip and dab it until you have ants stuck to the Q-tip," said the Vector Control guy.

This wasn't sounding so good, given that the same ants had snatched away my hand shovel earlier. But I'm a man, and I went forth. I trapped several of them on the gooey Q-tip.

Vector Control was pleased. "Great! Now drop the Q-tip in a plastic baggie and put that in your freezer for 15 minutes to kill them." In they went, next to some frozen broccoli.

Fifteen minutes later, I checked in. Vector Control wanted certainty. "Are they dead? Do you see any movement?" I assured him that nothing moved in the baggie o' death.

"Okay, now mail the baggie to this address." He gave me their top-secret Vector Control P.O. Box number, and I did as he said. First-class, all the way.

A couple of days later, our little street became a scene from *Ghostbusters*. A pickup truck with a special "Fire Ant Control" logo showed up. Little flags were planted in our lawn, as well as the closest neighbors'. Vector Control operatives sprayed all of our lawns with who-knows-what-and-if-you-did-we'd-have-to-kill-you spray.

The ants went away, and the lawns lived. I'm still not sure it wasn't just a weird dream.

Digging Around

You think the Fire Ant Busters are bizarre? Raising an autistic kid can require some weird tools and tactics.

"Fidgets" are one weapon. Pieces of tubing, paper, cloth, and all kinds of other material give the kid something to shake, rattle 'n' roll instead of shattering coffee mugs or tearing down curtains and shades.

"Redirection" produces an array of coded phrases that replace normal commands. "Are you ready to be calm?" takes the place of "Shut up before I come over there and …"

"How about come sit with Mom?" is the code for "Oh, my God, get away from that power tool!"

And the kids learn the dark arts and begin to apply them.

They come up with their own phrases:

"Do you want to go to the grass?" was Joey's way of saying, "I'm getting frustrated, and if you don't do something, I will harm people and property." Joey learned that phrase at school, where the teacher would offer him a walk around the sports field when he was agitated.

Then there's "Leave it," which means, "Oh, wait, that was for the dog, not the kid." Never mind.

Fertilizer

Jesus teaches us that things that sound bizarre and go against our intuitions can prove to be for the best. Not unlike catching fire ants on a Q-tip or speaking softly to Joey in situations that demand a shout. For example, Jesus goes completely against our normal assumptions when he says, "I am the vine; you are the branches. If you remain in me and I in you, you will bear much fruit; apart from me you can do nothing" (John 15:5 NIV).

What strange strategy is this? Shouldn't we be self-reliant, up by our own bootstraps, stiff-upper-lipped, soldiering on, etc.? I mean, come on, Jesus, I have the weight of the world on my shoulders here. There's a ton to get done, and it's all on me. I've got no time to "remain" or, as another translation says, "abide." It's go, go, go in my world.

But you're saying it's "Tim's world" only to the extent that I turn it into that, aren't you? It's your world, really, and I'm just one of the parts of it that you love and tend in every moment. And you want me to let you have more of your world back from my clutches and my worries, huh?

That's a strange approach, Jesus. It means to rely on your strength rather than my own. But mine seems to run out so quickly, and you—you've been at work forever.

Maybe I need to let you redirect me.

XXIV. SPRINKLER BLOW OUT AND WHATEVER THE OPPOSITE OF THAT IS

Another South Dakota discovery was the "sprinkler blow out." No, it's not a big sale on sprinkler stuff. It's having a guy come around before winter sets in to turn off the water to the sprinkler system and blow it out with nitrogen.

This is so there's no possible liquid left in the pipes because, in the winter, any water left in there will freeze, expand, and burst the pipes. And then it's either spend lots of money on repair or just say, "Okay, sun, when you come back in the summer, the lawn's all yours for a barbecue."

So around October every year, we call the sprinkler-blow-out guy to come do his thing. We haul the lawn hose into the garage and put insulated stuff over the outside faucets. Anything to do with outdoor water is shut down, covered up, or blown out.

And so it is until April when we call the guy again to come … uh… un-blow out? De-blow out? Blow in? Well, whatever he does to get the water flowing and the sprinklers running again for spring, summer, and fall.

Both routines are happy. The fall blowout means yard work is about to end for the winter months. The spring turn on means that winter is over. Good stuff, either way.

Digging Around

We all need happy routines in life. For people living with autism, structure is even more important. We have a sweet routine with Joey every Saturday. In the mornings, he has donuts from a local market's bakery. For dinner, he gets a freshly tossed pizza from their deli department.

He looks forward to this. As he's grown and has become more capable of anticipating future events, we see him lighting up as Friday comes, and he knows the next day will be donut and pizza time.

We tried to make Saturday a family restaurant outing, but he wasn't enjoying that. He wanted the donut and pizza routine at home. So we get some takeout for ourselves and delight together in Joey's laid-back weekend.

As we approach the time when Joey will move out of our house to live in a group home, we think that pizza at our place will continue as a routine when we pick him up for a weekly visit.

We will look forward to his moving out of the home and growing as an adult. But we will also look forward to continuing some sweet routines of the years we've shared under the same roof.

Fertilizer

God's universe includes rhythms and routines that carry us along. From the light and dark of day and night to the cycles of seasons and the passing of years, we are creatures who experience so much of our reality in these patterns. "And God said, 'Let there be lights in the vault of the sky to separate the day from the night, and let them serve as signs to mark sacred times, and days and years, and let them be lights in the vault of the sky to give light on the earth.' And it was so" (Genesis 1:14-15 NIV).

Because we are made in the image of God, we have the freedom and power to build special rhythms and routines into our lives. Anniversaries of all kinds, an annual fishing trip with friends, a couple's weekly date night, anticipation of a favorite TV show, and other such happenings beyond number are a powerful part of who we are.

The Creator of all gave the rhythms and routines to "give light upon the earth." May we be blessed to discover routines that brighten our days. And may we find routines that light up the lives of those in our care.

XXV. THE EVERGREEN

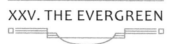

Our South Dakota front yard boasts a huge evergreen tree. A giant Christmas tree is one way to describe it.

I didn't appreciate evergreens until I moved here. Sure, they were pretty and made me think of forests. But I wasn't accustomed to all of the trees and plants (even the grass in the yard) going bare and dormant for the winter months. So seeing that big green life standing tall over the autumn brown and winter white made me understand the "ever" part of its name.

And the life shining from that evergreen isn't just its own. It is where all kinds of birds make nests, including the gorgeous Northern Cardinals that we love to see on our feeders. The rabbits retreat under the evergreen to hide out from our dog, who gets a good workout running around the tree in her vain efforts to catch them. Squirrels use it as a launch pad to spring onto the bird feeder to steal seeds.

Because the evergreen is there, many other creatures can live.

Digging Around

There's another Tim. No, not some symbolic dark side of myself. He's the first son with whom Melissa and I were blessed; he's Joey's older brother.

I've gone back and forth about putting him in this book. He has his own life. He's not just some sidekick character or an amusing interloper like the dog.

But autism changed his family and exerted considerable

influence over his life.

I won't recapitulate all of the perils that Joey posed to Melissa and me, except to say that Tim put up with all of the same, and had to do so as a child.

This whole book explored the demands of caregiving, so I won't recap, except to say that Tim had to deal with all of them, as well as his own life's needs and challenges. We missed his high school graduation ceremony because Joey was sick or in a mood or whatever it was that night that made it impossible to go.

There's no way to do justice to Tim's place in this story in a single chapter. It would require a book of its own. Like the evergreen, he's stood through all of the seasons.

And even with all the costs to himself over the years, he stood before a judge with us and committed to being Joey's guardian when Melissa and I will no longer be able. Like that tree that shelters the birds and bunnies, Tim stands ready to shelter Joey.

I'm pretty sure he'll be more of an evergreen than a blooming idiot.

Fertilizer

Another blooming idiot confession: I call that tree in the front yard an evergreen because I've never bothered to ask if it is a spruce, a fir, or whatever. It is just there, and I don't do much of anything for it except delight in it.

Jesus was honored and comforted by a woman whose name the Bible never reveals. But God delights in her. Jesus said, "Truly I tell you, wherever the gospel is preached throughout the world, what she has done will also be told, in memory of her" (Mark 14:9 NIV).

Since I've already compared our son Tim to our nameless tree, why not compare him to a nameless girl? He wasn't Joey's official caregiver, yet even without that title assigned, he stepped up for caregiving situations that God placed in his path, like the woman who had no obligation but who chose to care for Jesus.

He's been a caregiver to Joey, from feeding and bathing his brother to entertaining him with music. He's been a caregiver to Melissa and me, taking on tasks without being asked to make all of our lives easier. As a teenager, he would throw in Joey's laundry when doing his own, saving Mom and Dad from one more chore.

Jesus reveals that those who show kindness and honor to others in the midst of all of life's demands and choices are part of the eternal good news of God's world-changing love. Like evergreens, they stand as shelters for those shivering in a cold world and shade for those weakened by its heat.

Caregivers, and those in our care, can't endure without such people. And we've been blessed to have one in our son and brother: Tim.

XXVI. A MOVING STORY

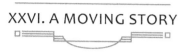

When we moved from Southern California to South Dakota, we knew that Melissa's gardenias would not survive such a journey. Yet we didn't want to leave them untended.

Joey had a music therapist who came to our house, and we knew she was a fan of those fragrant white flowers. So Melissa offered them to her.

The gardenias had quite the send-off. The therapist came over with her husband and their big dog. She did a last music session with Joey, and we had a farewell party.

The time came to say goodbye, and it wasn't easy. It was hard to leave kind people who bettered Joey's life, and it was a special tug at Melissa's heart to give away those gardenias. It took years to get those flowers to flourish, and now she had to give away what she'd tended with so much time, effort, and attention.

As a man, I find physical tasks to be the perfect escape from emotional scenes. So I set myself to toting the gardenias in their large terra-cotta pots into the back of their station wagon that would take the flowers to their new home.

The empty spots where they used to be were too much for me to look at, so as the music therapist drove away, I found other tasks to fuss over.

Digging Around

Giving away gardenias hardly compares to the "giveaway" in our future: Joey is now on a waiting list to move into a group residence. It is uncomfortable to think about looking into his bedroom, just down the hall from ours, and seeing an empty space. Like Melissa's gardenias, he's grown in beautiful ways. And the time is coming to let him go.

Oh, sure, we've longed for the day. The years of effort and the limitations placed on our lives have seemed like a jail sentence at times. But he's someone precious to us, and this is going to be hard. We worry about how he will do without us, despite every other caregiver reassuring us that their kid adjusted from living under Mom and Dad to thriving in a new setting.

We know they're telling the truth. We know that we do a lot for Joey that he will learn to do for himself. Imitating peers in adult living will be more influential than enduring instructions from Mom and Dad.

But I sense that Melissa and I will both need to be busy with all kinds of distracting tasks for several days after we move him to a new home.

Fertilizer

We have so many ways to stay connected today. Social media like Facebook and communication systems like Skype let us hear and see one another in real time, any time. Who knows what new stuff will be available by the time you read this? Facebook might be like cave paintings in the not too distant future.

Even with all of our technology, partings remain "sweet sorrow." Bonds that have provided joy, comfort, and dependability are released. No matter how reverently or tenderly that takes place, we feel the loss. Pictures and voices are partial. They don't bring us touch, fragrance or any of the other sensual qualities of those who've gone away.

There's a moving farewell scene in the Bible, set in a time where physical distance did not have the compensations of audio/visual devices.

> In everything I did, I showed you that by this kind
> of hard work we must help the weak, remembering

the words the Lord Jesus himself said: "It is more blessed to give than to receive." When Paul had finished speaking, he knelt down with all of them and prayed. They all wept as they embraced him and kissed him. What grieved them most was his statement that they would never see his face again. Then they accompanied him to the ship. (Acts 20:35-38 NIV)

Paul's painful farewell is prefaced by the reminder that in Jesus, giving away is a source of blessedness: deep, abiding joy.

This requires a leap of faith. Looked at with our human eyes, letting go and giving away provoke feelings of loss, uncertainty, fear, and maybe even some powerful resentment. We miss what we had; we feel the passage of time and our own mortality, and we worry about how others will do without us.

The leap of faith is to trust that all lives are in the care of God. What we've given away will be tended to by God, who receives our efforts as a precious offering. The relationships we enjoy are a gift, and if we have faith in God, we can pass those gifts along, knowing that they will be in the best possible care.

In *The Book of Common Prayer*, there are excellent words to offer "for those we love:"

"Almighty God, we entrust all who are dear to us to thy never-failing care and love, for this life and the life to come, knowing that thou art doing for them better things than we can desire or pray for; through Jesus Christ our Lord. *Amen.*"

XXVII. WITH THE BEST OF INTENTIONS

On the anniversary of something or other, a friend sent me flowers at my office. I was touched that a special event in my life had been recognized, and I fiddled around with stuff on a bookshelf and file cabinet tops to find just the right place to display the bouquet.

As a blooming idiot well aware of my limitations, I made sure the vase had plenty of water. I made sure the shades were up to let in some sun. At the end of the day, I went merrily home, savoring the aroma of the flowers as I locked the office door.

The next morning, the flowers were deader than dead. They looked like they'd been outdoors through several months of winter.

My office is in an add-on to the original building, an addition that the owners describe as "practical and economical." You got it: cheap, as in poorly insulated. So when the temperature dropped overnight, frigid air got to the flowers.

A blooming idiot outcome, but not for lack of good intentions.

Digging Around

Melissa and I sometimes think about "if only" scenarios for Joey. "If only the schools had provided this or that service to him at this or that time in his life." "If only we'd known about X before he was Y and that led to Z."

When it comes to Joey, I am confident that our intentions

been the best. But turning intentions into
on doesn't always happen, as I saw with that
ent in my office.

.. nen it came to negotiating his program with schools, we
can point to times when we probably didn't assert ourselves
enough, trusted the "experts," and wound up with less than
Joey needed.

Other times, we might have been too zealous, turned
people off, and, you guessed it, wound up with less than Joey
needed.

Then there have been our own limitations as flesh-and-
blood human beings. We purchased materials to use with
Joey, but then we gave up on them after not much effort.
We passed on activities that might have been at least fun, if
not constructive, because we anticipated the hassle that Joey
would give us if we tried.

On balance, I'm not ashamed. We've done well by Joey,
both by our own appraisal of his life, the assessment of others
close to us, and his own happiness and health. But that doesn't
deny the fact that we've had plenty of failures along the way.

Fertilizer

A realistic look at human life sees tragic imperfection, and
many of our failures get no "do over." A moment or a season
passes, and the opportunity to "get it right" is gone.

Moral failure, in particular, clings to us, either via
consequences or by the fact that we have hard-wired character
flaws that keep the failures coming. If we have a conscience
for ourselves and a heart for others, this reality can cause deep
grief, even despair.

The message of Christian faith is that our imperfection is
not the final word. We need not deny it. In fact, we jeopardize
our souls if we do, but if we own it honestly, and turn to God
for help, we find mercy.

But if we walk in the light, as he is in the light, we
have fellowship with one another, and the blood of

Jesus, his Son, purifies us from all sin. If we claim to be without sin, we deceive ourselves and the truth is not in us. If we confess our sins, he is faithful and just and will forgive us our sins and purify us from all unrighteousness. (I John 1:7-9 NIV)

We are cleansed by the blood of Jesus, the Son of God. He was perfect, without flaw, always doing the will of God. He offers to God what we cannot give, and he offers it on our behalf.

As I wrap up this bundle of thoughts, I realize that they are imperfect. They're an example of my blooming idiocy, a bunch of stunted plants and weeds. I might have said things in better ways, or come up with better examples, or put less of myself in some parts and more of myself in others.

The same can be said of Joey's life, my marriage to Melissa, and any other aspect of my life. Imperfections abound, some of them from simple limitations, and some of them from deep-seeded character flaws that are like weeds, always coming back no matter how much I try to get rid of them.

But I keep on. I do not despair because it is not my blooming idiocy but the blood of Jesus that cleanses and makes perfect my imperfectly offered life. God is faithful, just, and will never reject those who come to him through Jesus.

I pray that some who read this will discover this good news. You are loved by God, with all of the flaws and struggles that cling to your life as a caregiver. The only perfect offering has been made for you by Jesus on the cross.

So let me remind you of that little story from the start of this book:

Then [Jesus] told this parable: "A man had a fig tree growing in his vineyard, and he went to look for fruit on it but did not find any. So he said to the man who took care of the vineyard, 'For three years now I've been coming to look for fruit on this fig tree and haven't found any. Cut it down! Why should it use up the soil?' "'Sir,' the man replied, 'leave it alone for one more year, and I'll dig around it and fertilize it. If it bears fruit next year, fine! If not, then cut it down.'" (Luke 13:6-9 NIV)

When you're overwhelmed, Jesus says, "One more chance."
When you've failed, Jesus says, "One more chance."
When you're angry or resentful, Jesus says, "One more chance."

You see, he doesn't mean "only one more." He means "the next fresh start." And he's there to give "special attention and fertilizer." His Spirit and his Word are yours if you will embrace your blooming idiocy and let him take over the tending of your life and the lives in your care.

So, speaking of gardening stuff, I'll leave you with "watering." Here are words from Holy Baptism, through which lives are given to God through Jesus by the power of the Holy Spirit. If you're already baptized, reclaim the significance of it. It never "wore off." Jesus is with you. If you haven't been baptized, consider offering these words of faith and finding a Christian community to baptize and support you.

Question	Do you turn to Jesus Christ and accept him as your Savior?
Answer	I do.
Question	Do you put your whole trust in his grace and love?
Answer	I do.
Question	Do you promise to follow and obey him as your Lord?
Answer	I do.

(Book of Common Prayer, 1979)

If you can say this, you're a blooming idiot like me. But now the emphasis is on "blooming." Amen.

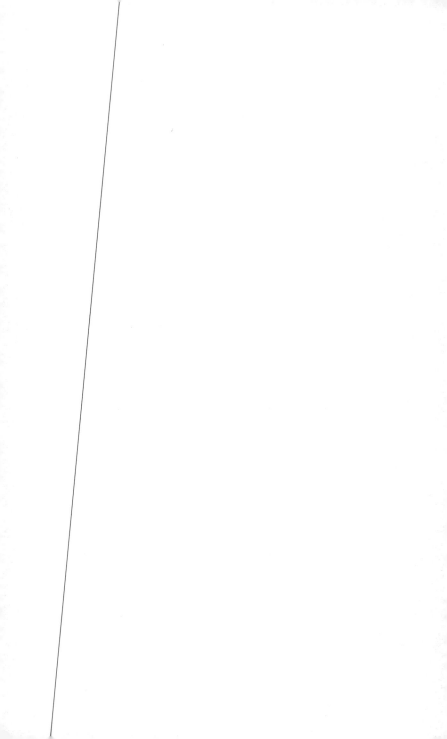

Made in the USA
Middletown, DE
31 January 2020